- Table of Contents -

Skeletal System
Muscular System
Nervous System
Endocrine System
Cardiovascular System
Lymphatic System
Respiratory System
Digestive System
Male Reproductive System
Female Reproductive System
Urinary System
Immune System
Integumentary System
Heart and Blood Circulation System

Upper Respiratory Tract Infection
Sinusitis
Tonsillitis
Laryngitis
Epiglottis
Lower Respiratory Tract Infection
Pneumonia
Bronchitis
Bronchiolitis
Tuberculosis
Croup
Asthma
Chronic Obstructive Pulmonary Disease (COPD)
Obstructive Sleep Apnea (OSA)
Cystic Fibrosis
Lung Cancer
Pulmonary Fibrosis
Sepsis
Bacteremia
Endocarditis
Pericarditis
High Blood Pressure
Coronary Artery Disease
Myocardial Infarction
Heart Failure
Cardiac Arrhythmia
Peripheral Artery Disease
Aortic Aneurysms
Deep Vein Thrombosis (DTV)
Pulmonary Embolism
Cardiomyopathy
Heart Valve Disease
Gastroenteritis
Peptic Ulcer Disease
Gastroesophageal Reflux Disease
Gastritis
Ulcerative Colitis (Inflammatory Bowel Disease : IBD)

Irritable Bowel Syndrome - IBS
Diverticulitis
Cirrhosis
Pancreatitis
Gallstones
Colorectal Cancer
Meningitis
Viral Encephalitis
Brain Abscess
Cerebral Malaria
Types of Brain Stroke
Alzheimer's Disease
Parkinson's Disease
Huntington's Disease
Multiple Sclerosis
Epilepsy
Amyotrophic Lateral Sclerosis (ALS)
Neuropathy
Urinary Tract Infection - UTI
Kidney Stones
Types of Incontinence
Benign Prostatic Hyperplasia
Prostatitis
Interstitial Cystitis
Erectile Dysfunction
Polycystic Kidney
Endometriosis
Pyelonephritis
Genital Herpes
Vaginal Thrush
Pelvic Inflammatory Diseases
Impetigo
Cellulite
Athlete's Foot
Ringworm
Three Kinds of Fungal Infections
Herpes Simples (Lips/Mouth)
Wart
Scabies
Candidiasis
Dental Caries (Tooth Decay)
Gingivitis
Periodontitis
Dental Abscess
Osteomyelitis
Septic Arthritis
Osteoarthritis
Rheumatoid Arthritis
Gout
Necrotizing Fasciitis
Osteoporosis

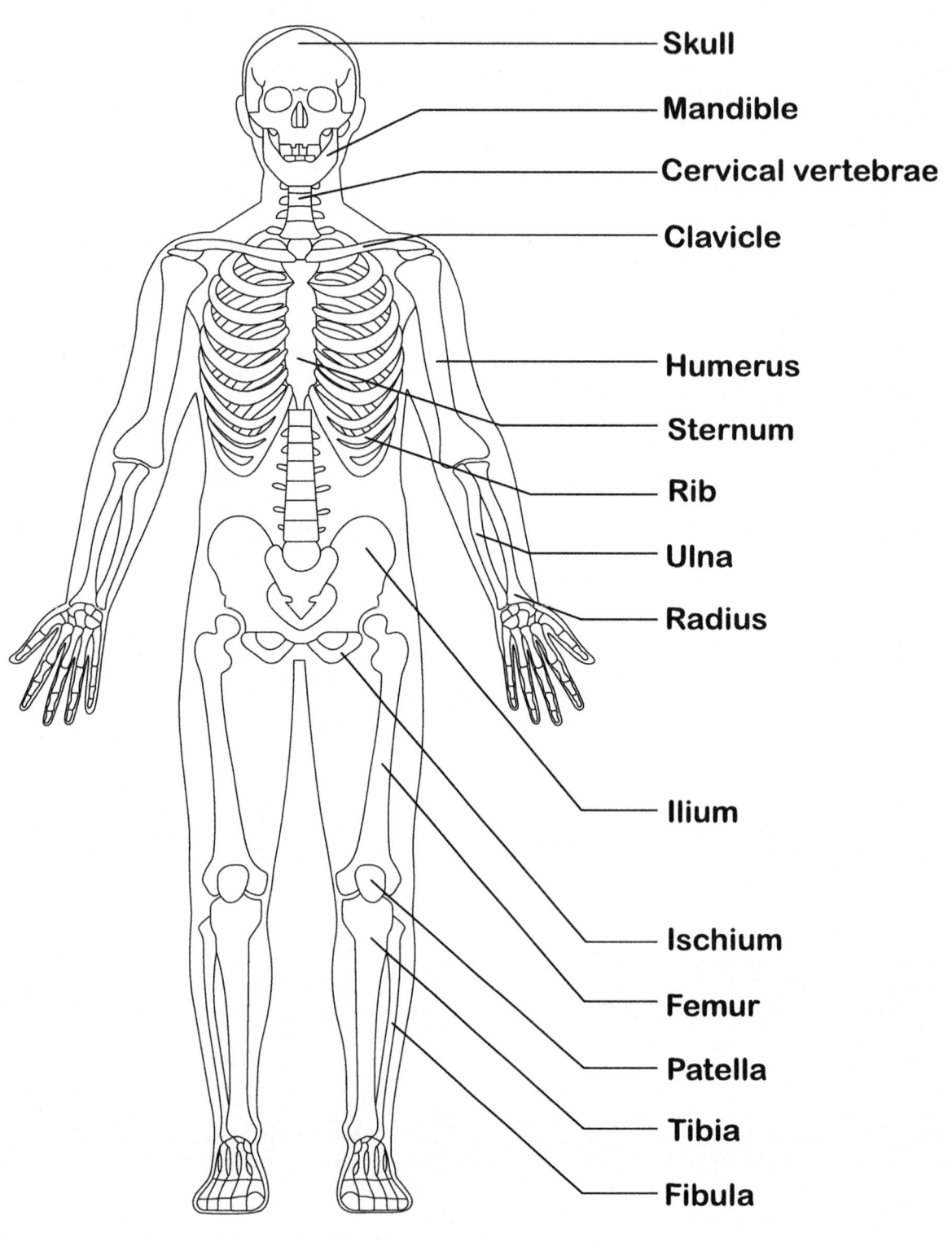

Skeletal System
Back

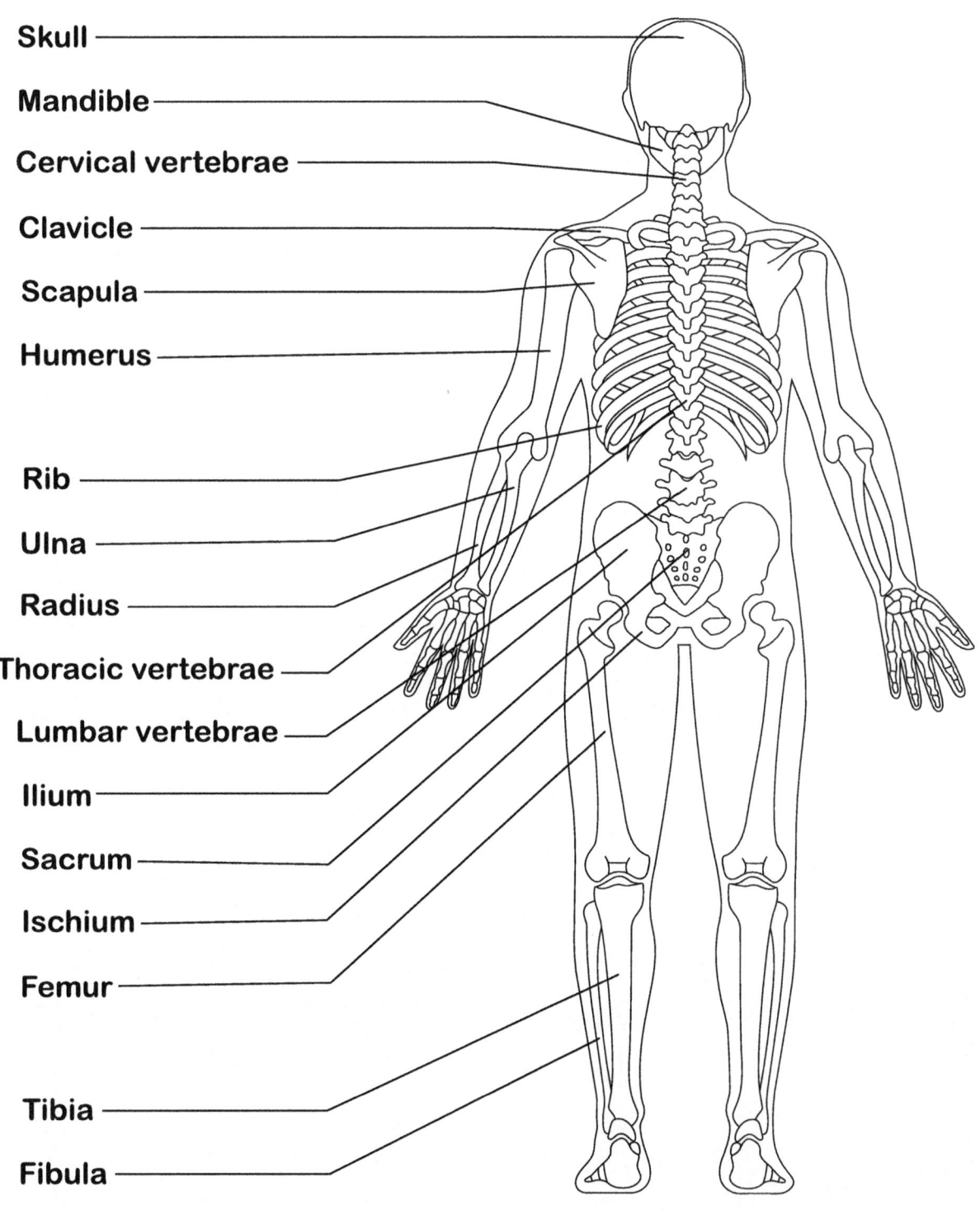

- Skull
- Mandible
- Cervical vertebrae
- Clavicle
- Scapula
- Humerus
- Rib
- Ulna
- Radius
- Thoracic vertebrae
- Lumbar vertebrae
- Ilium
- Sacrum
- Ischium
- Femur
- Tibia
- Fibula

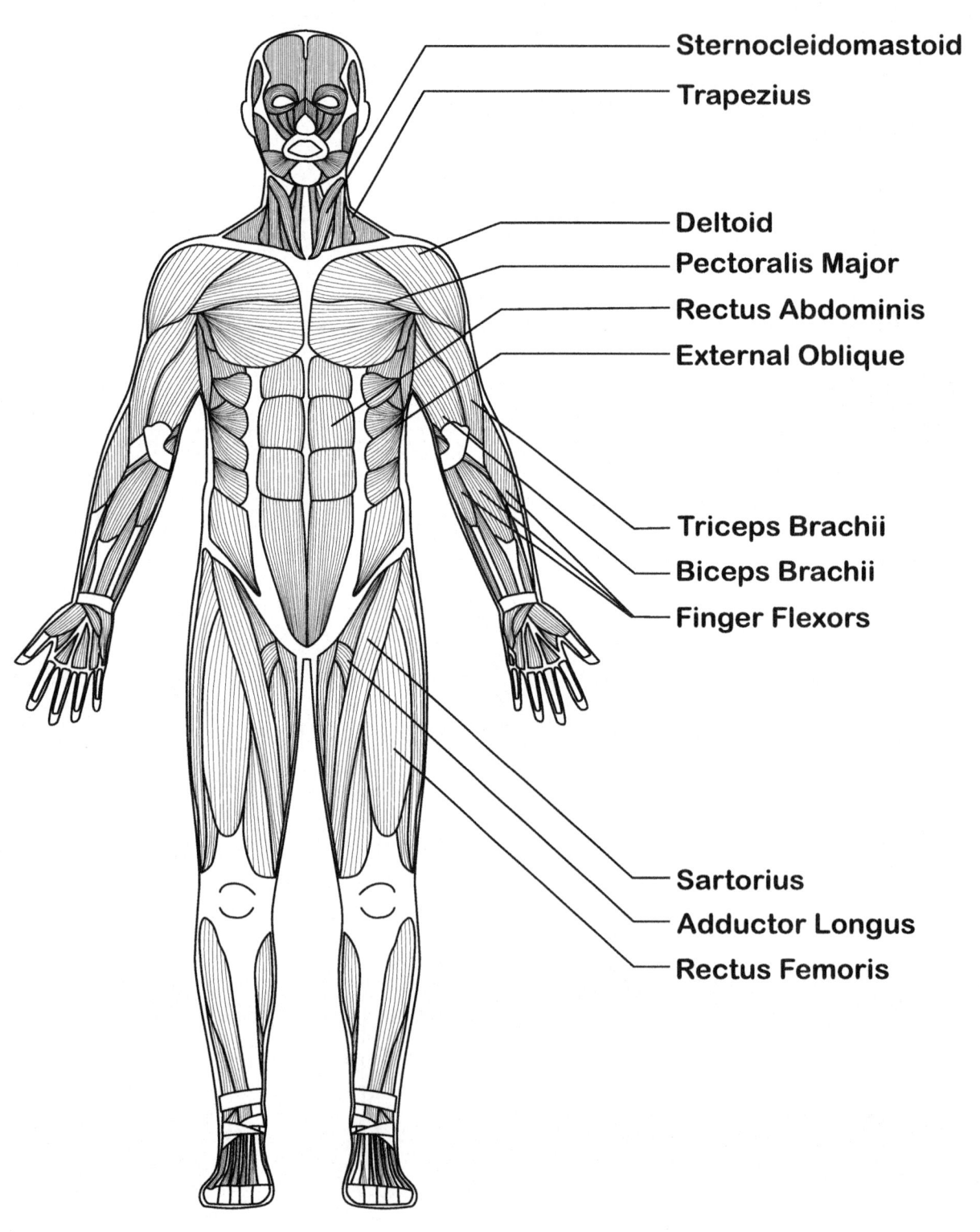

Muscular System
Back

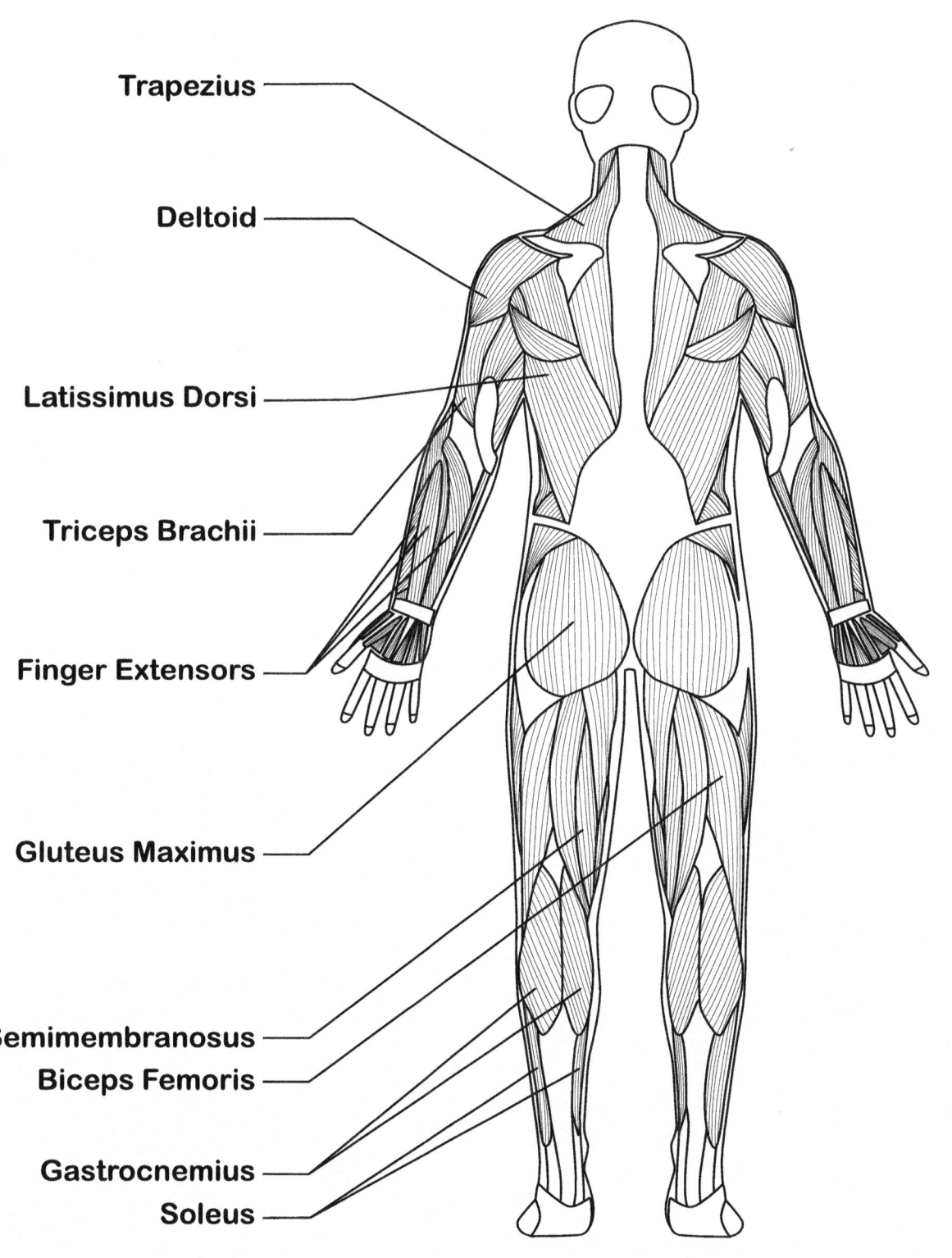

- Trapezius
- Deltoid
- Latissimus Dorsi
- Triceps Brachii
- Finger Extensors
- Gluteus Maximus
- Semimembranosus
- Biceps Femoris
- Gastrocnemius
- Soleus

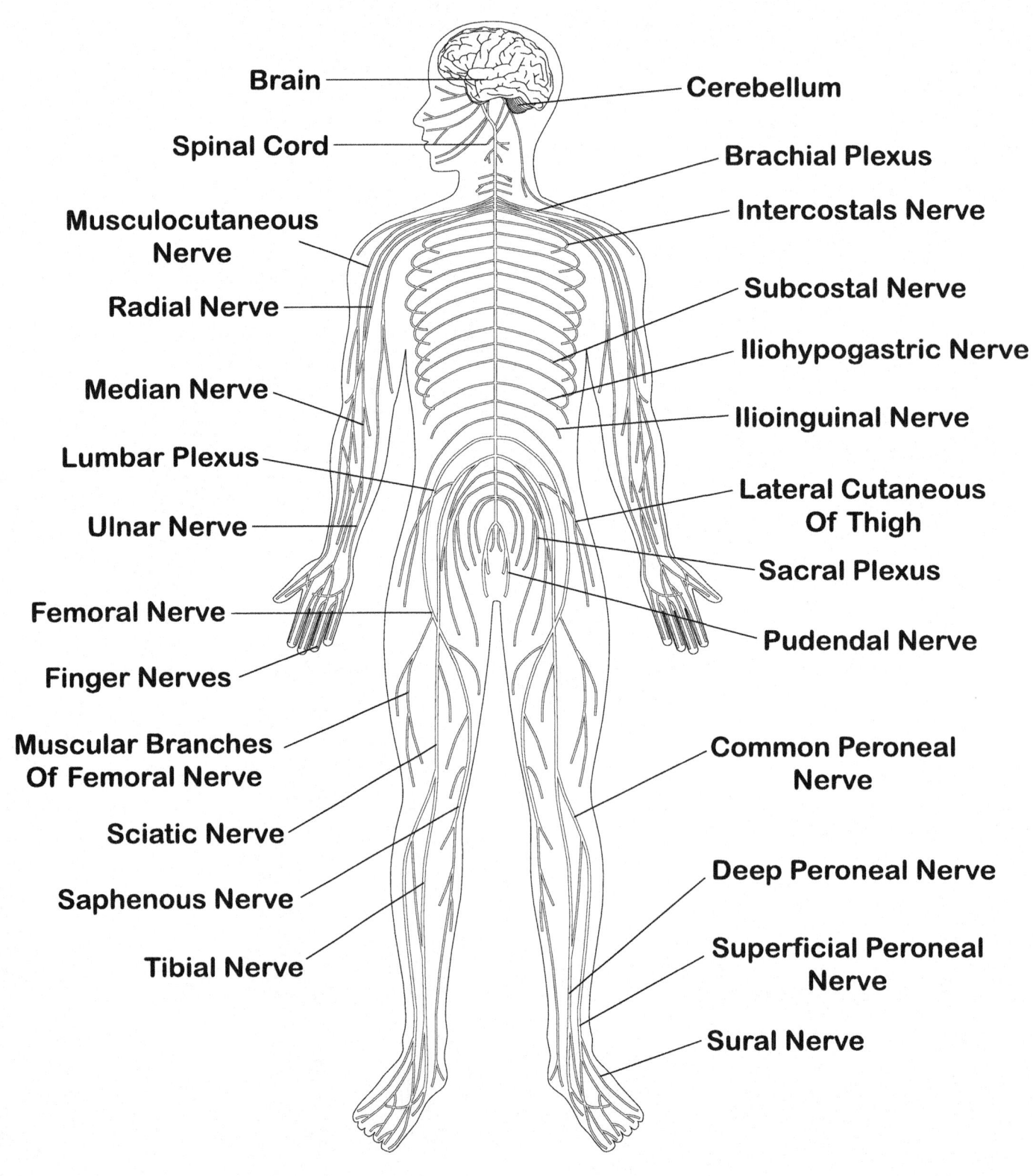

Endocrine System

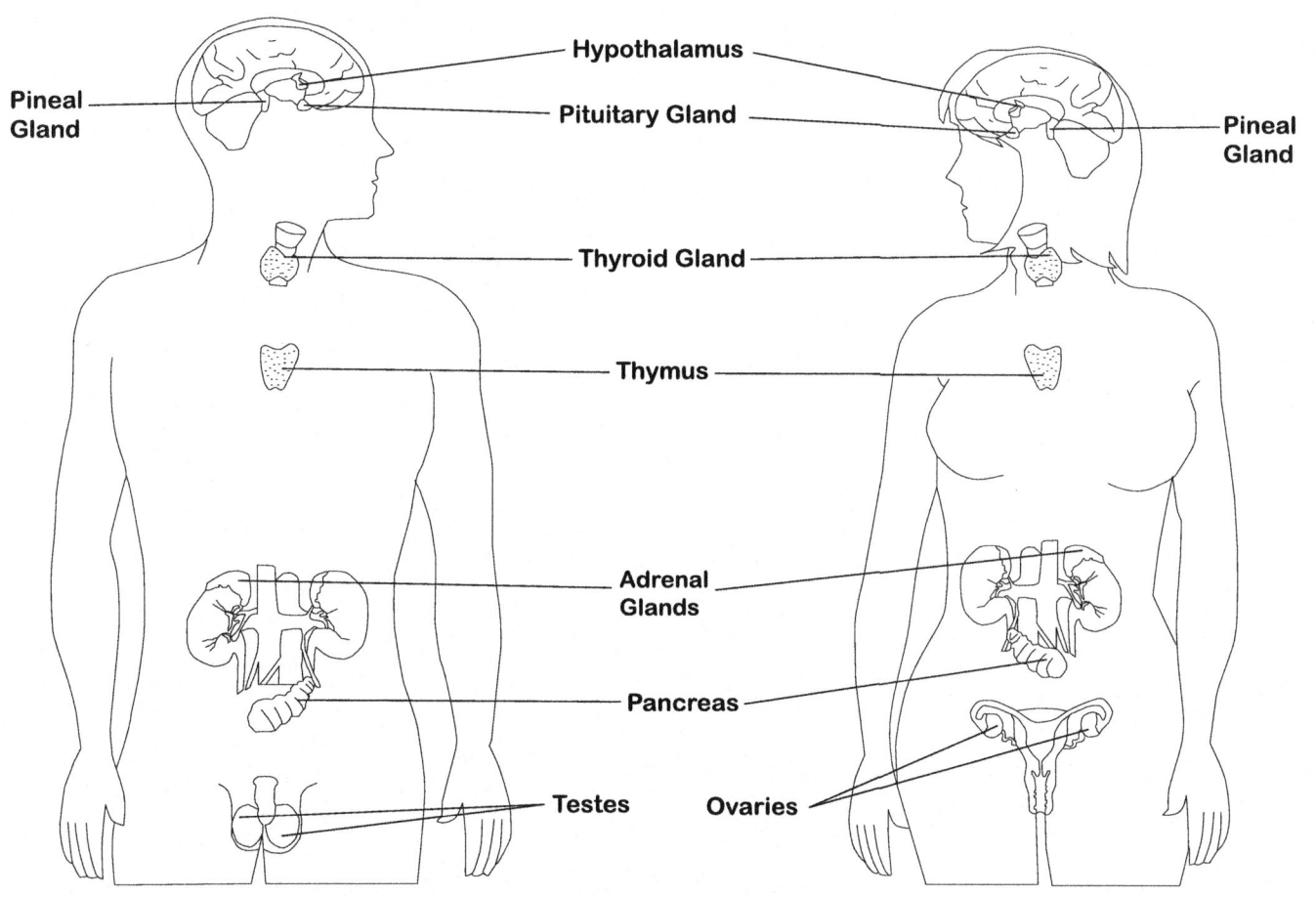

Cardiovascular System

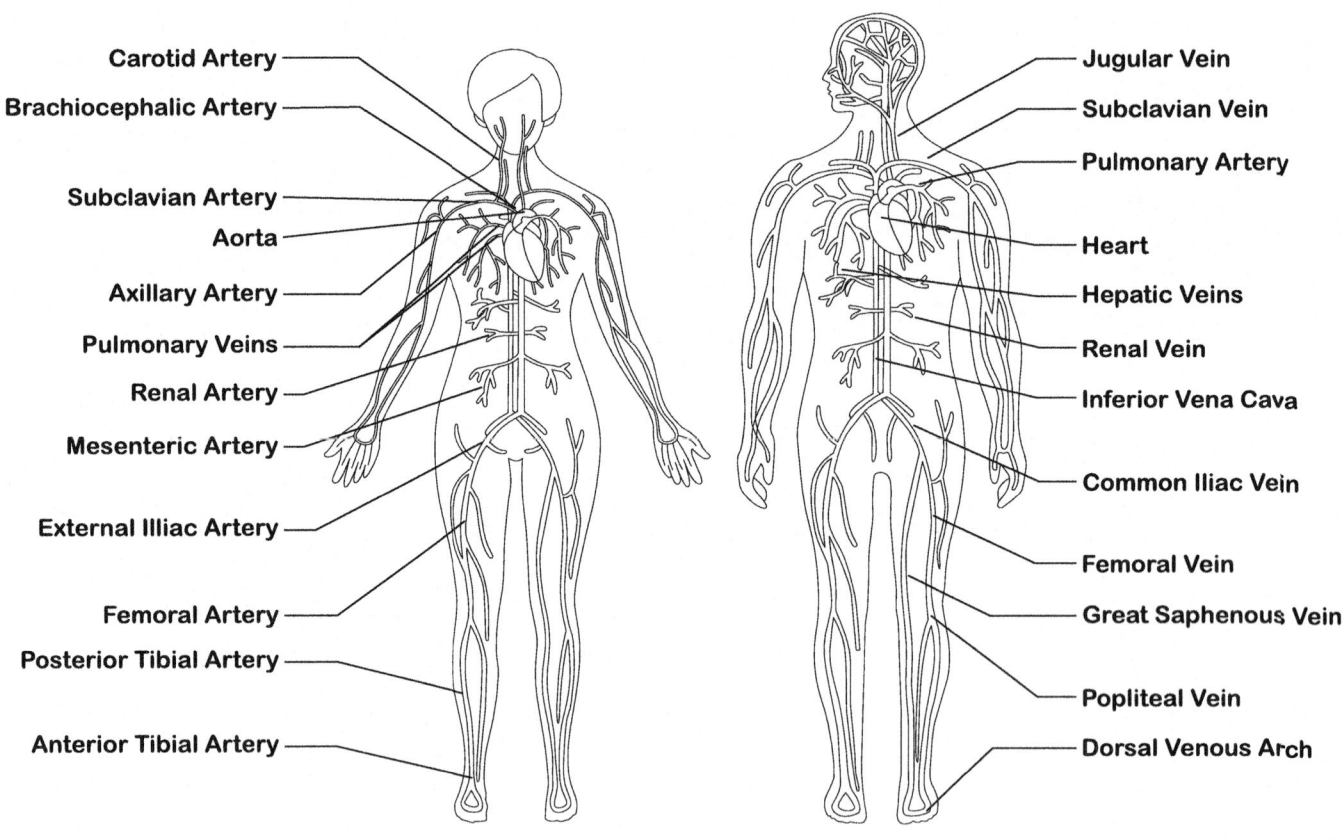

Lymphatic System

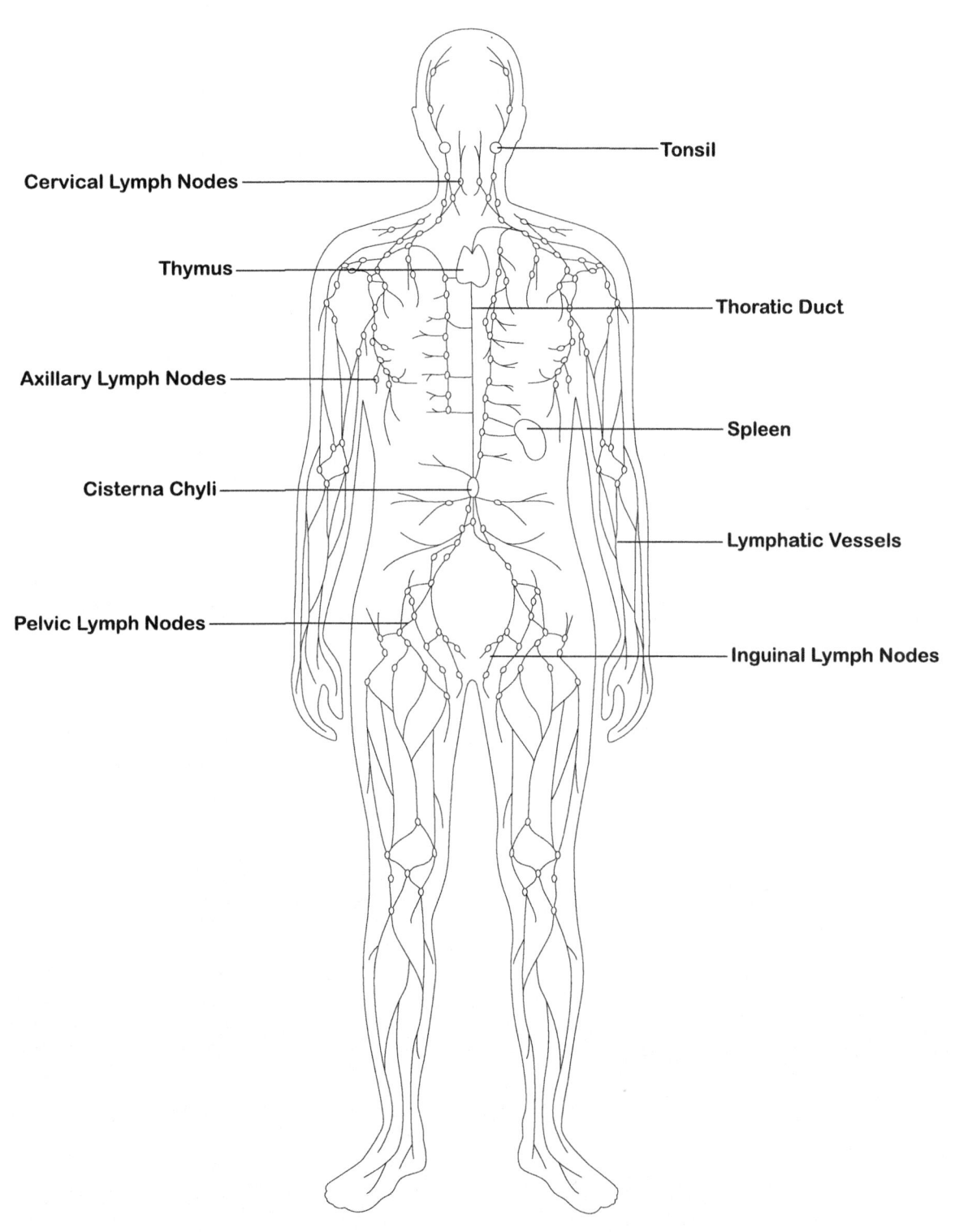

Respiratory System

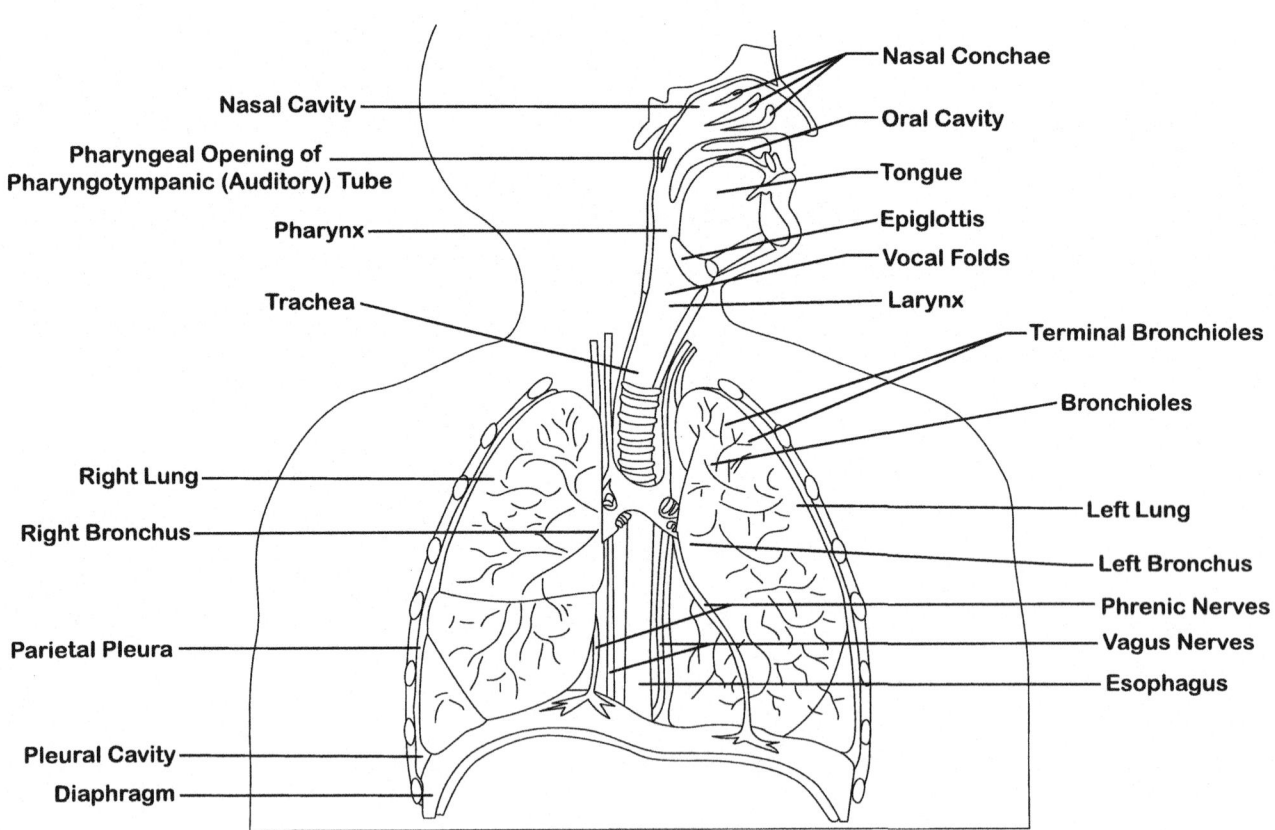

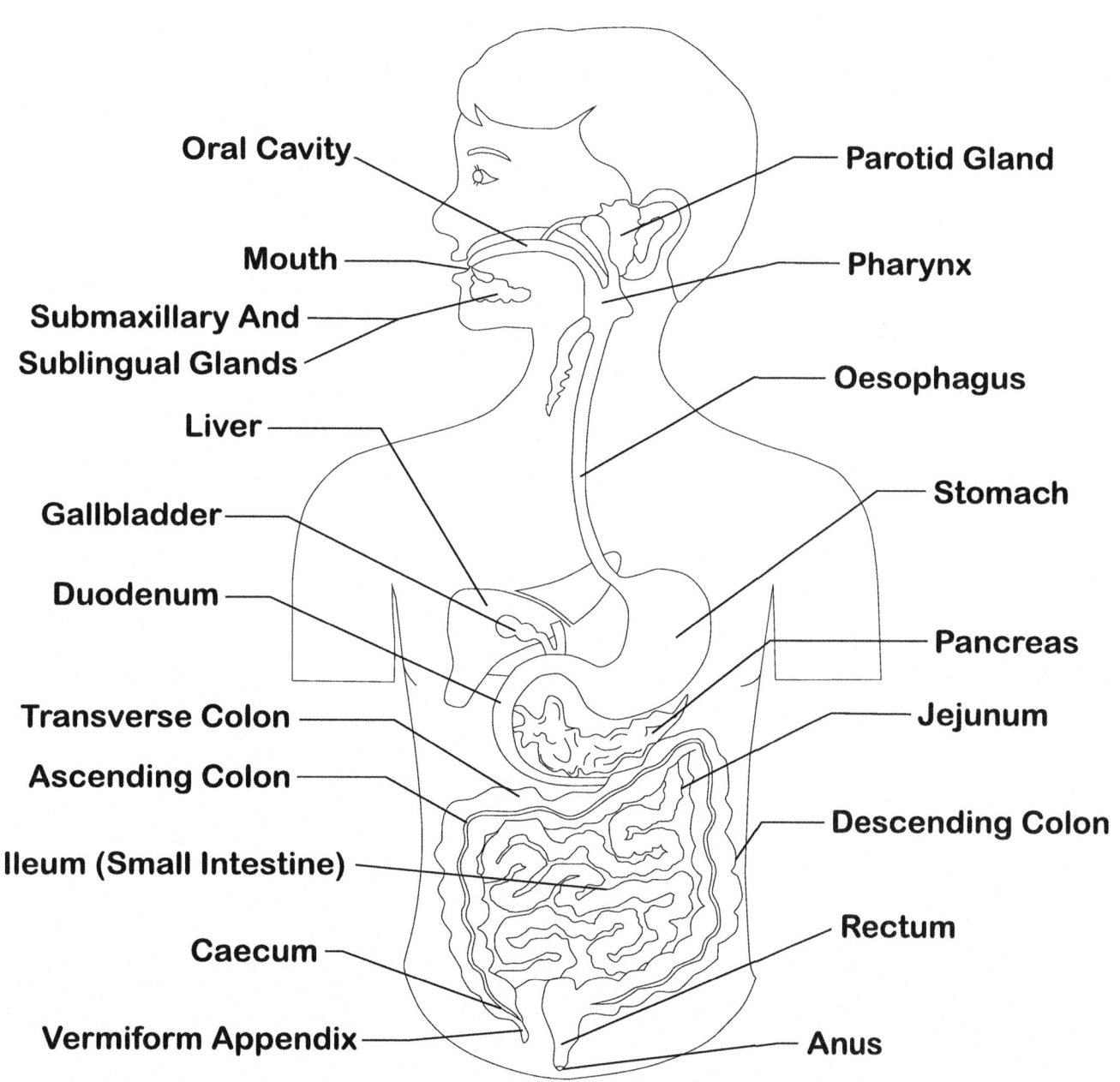

Male Reproductive System

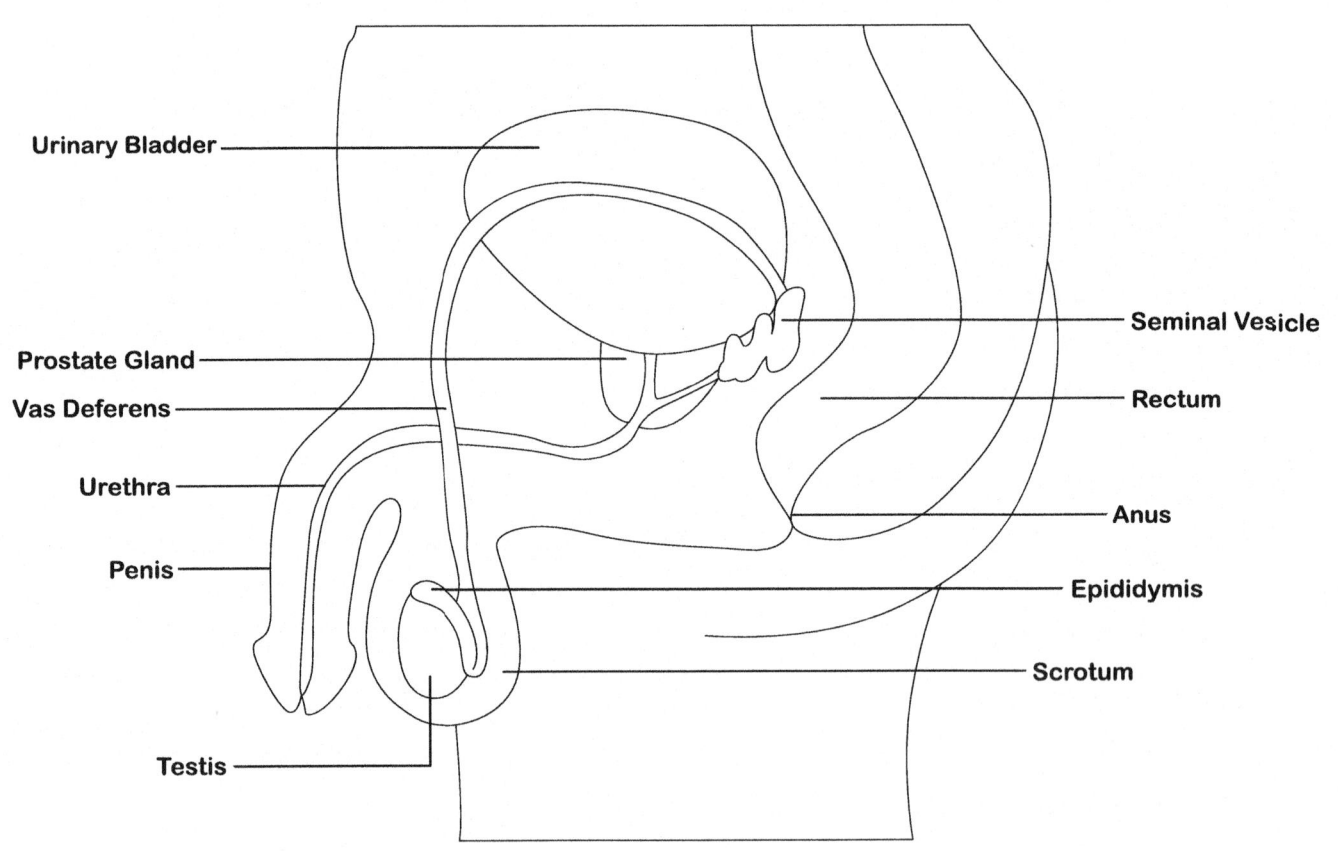

Female Reproductive System

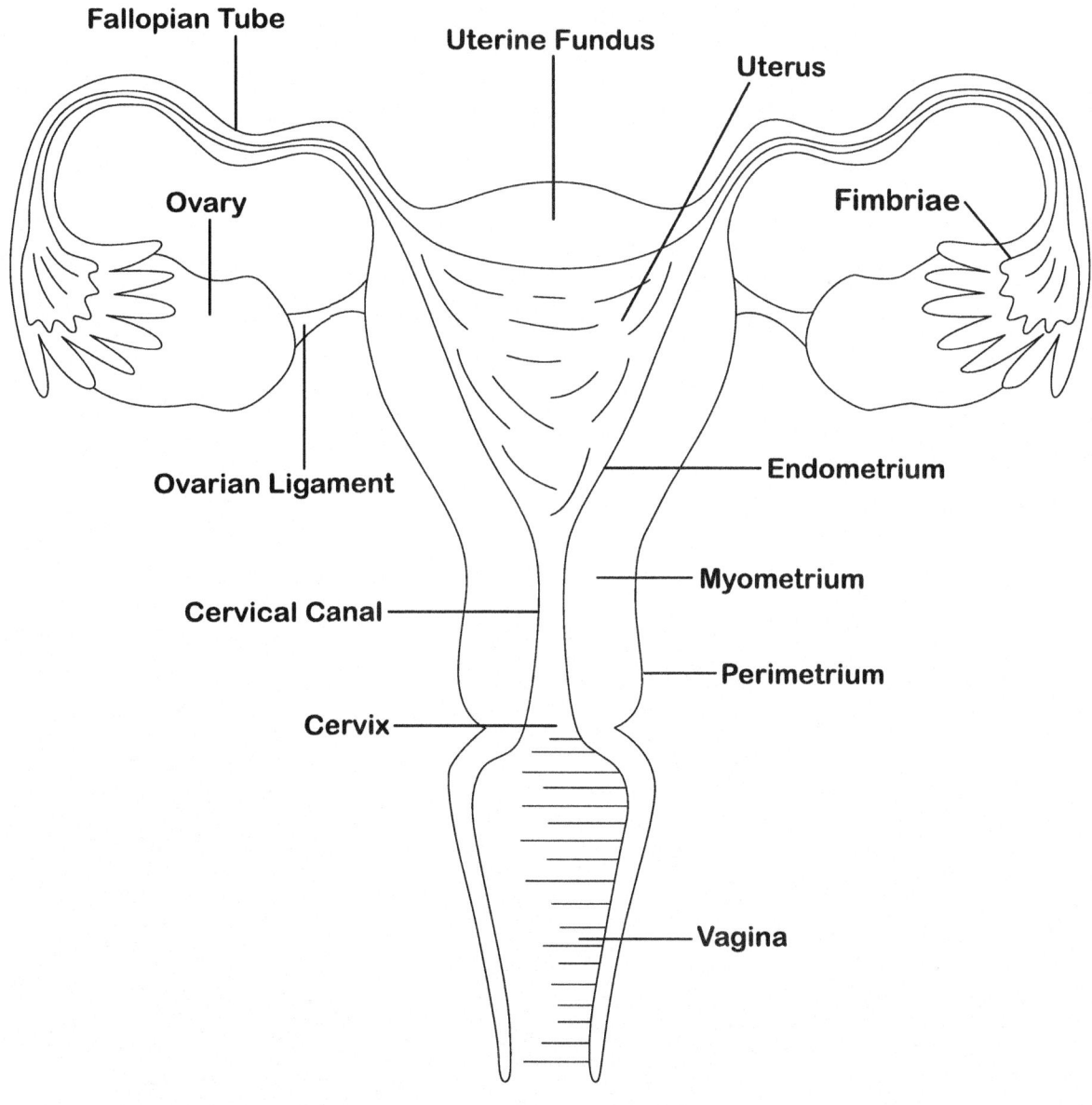

Urinary System
Urinary Tract

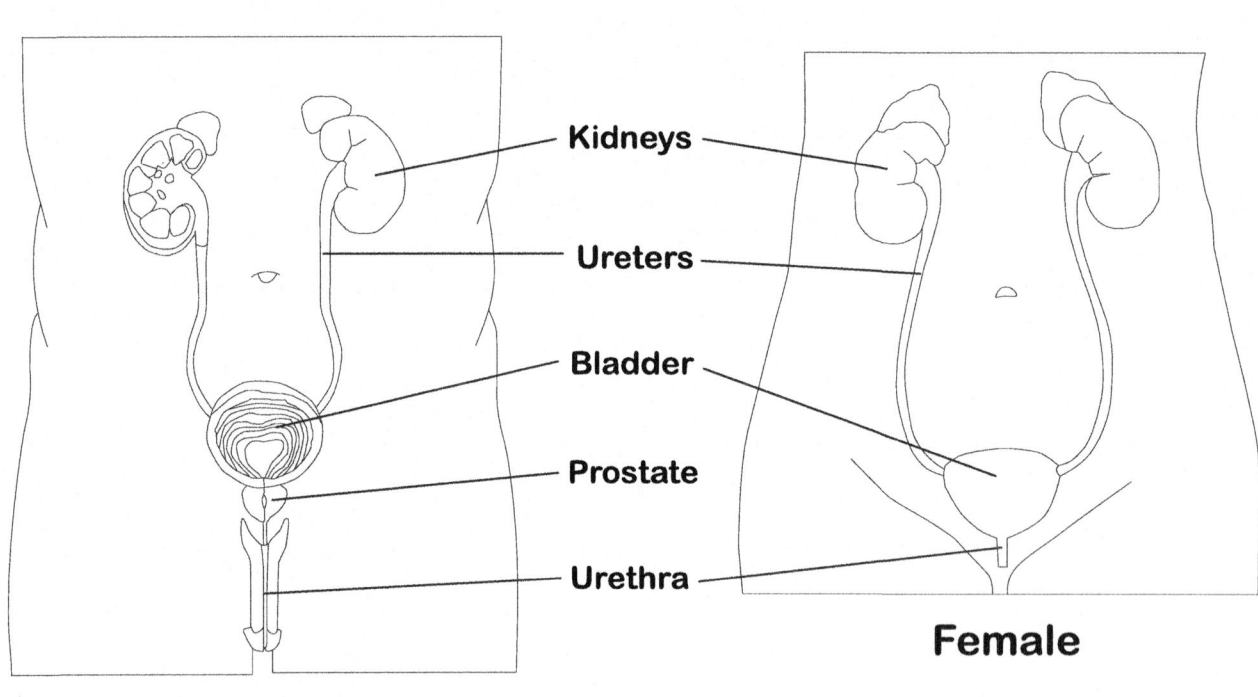

Male

Female

Immune System

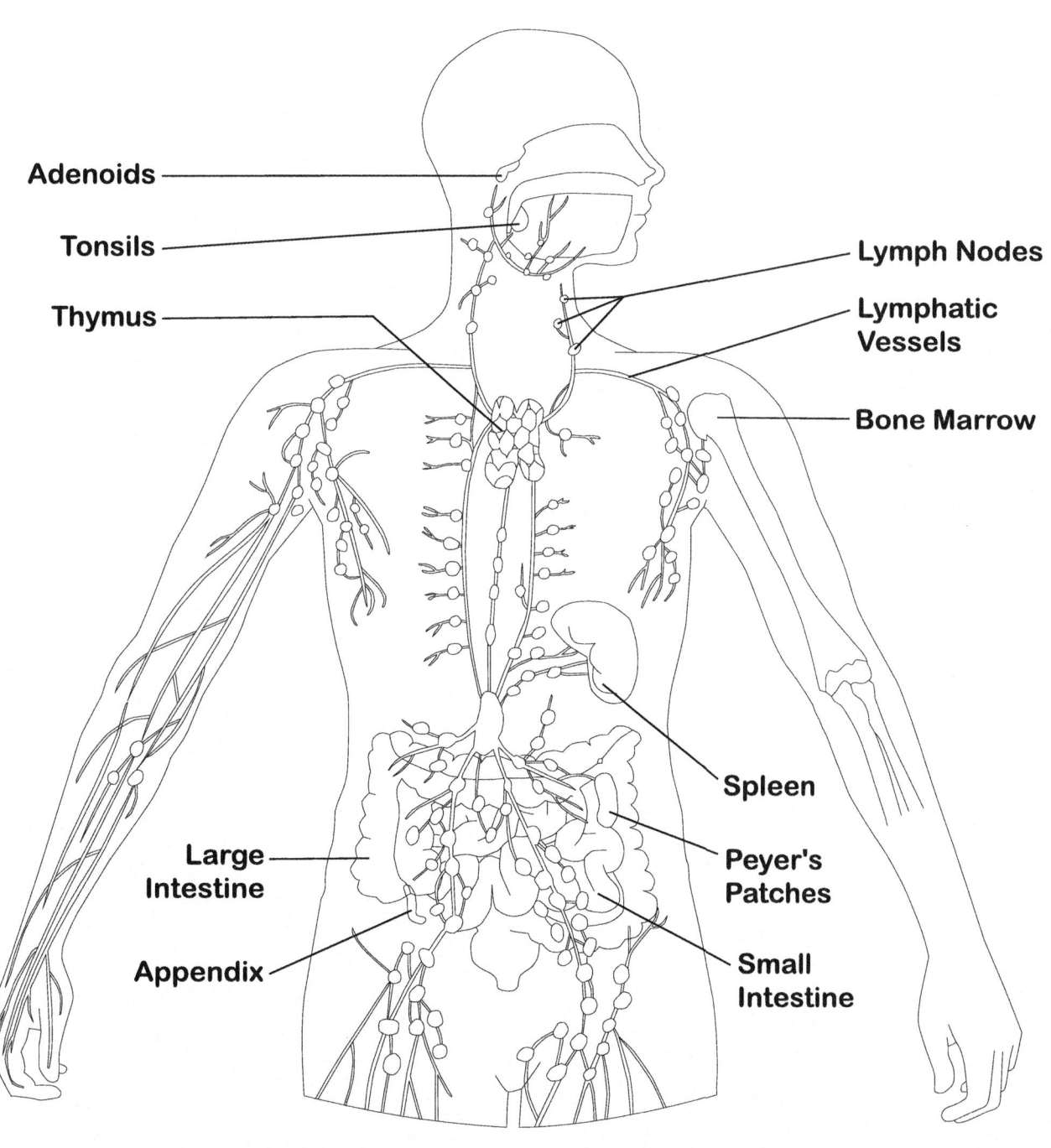

Integumentary System

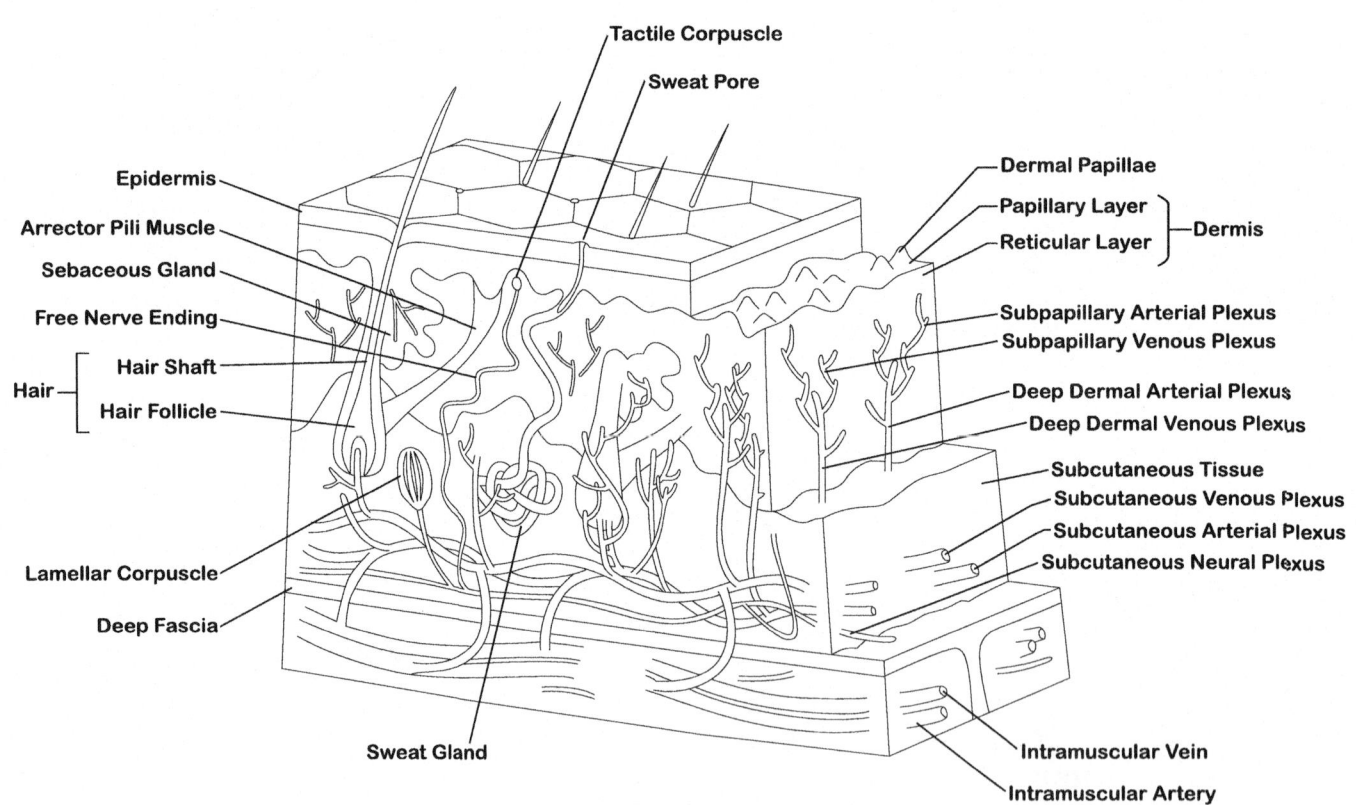

Heart and Blood Circulation System

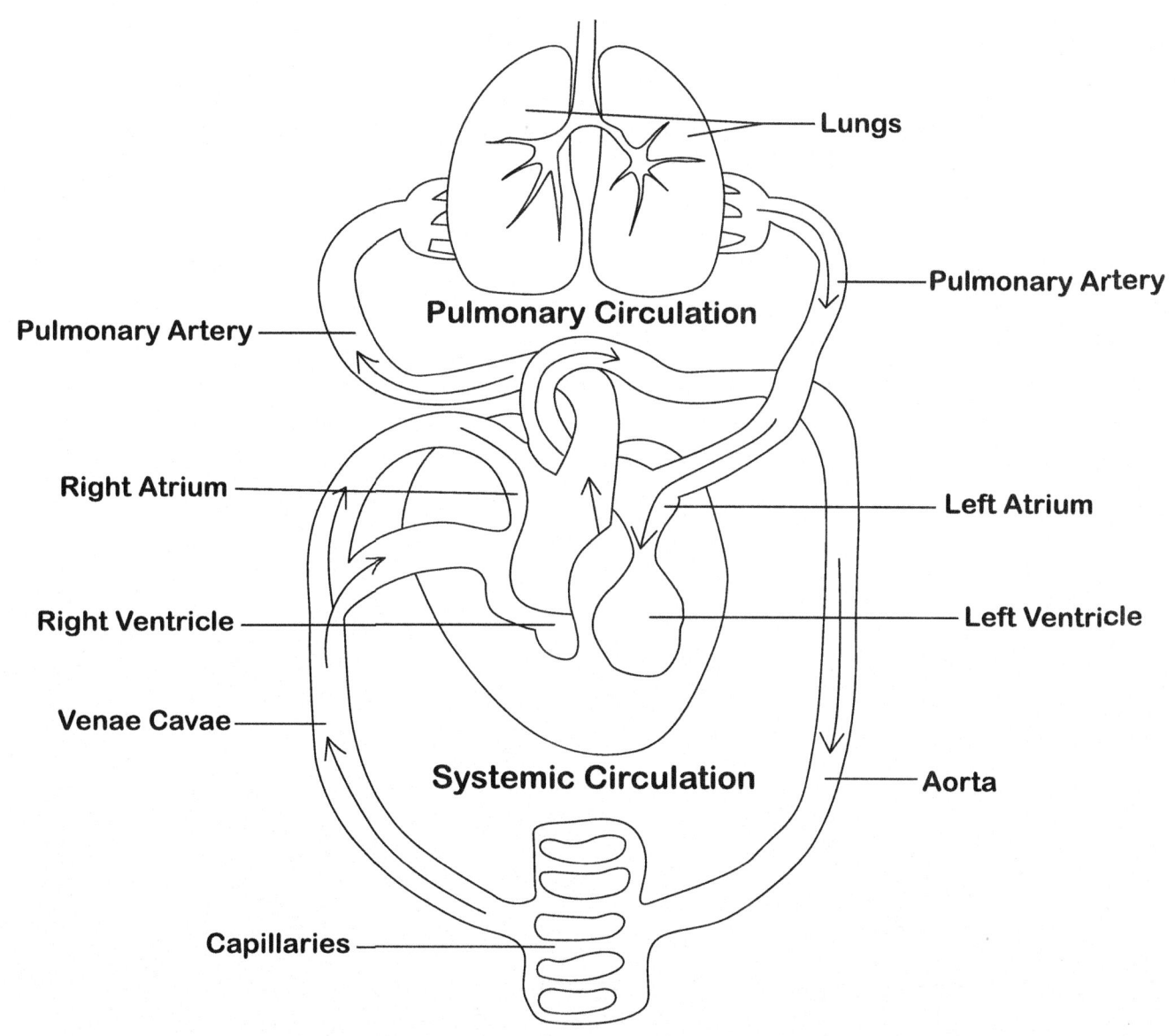

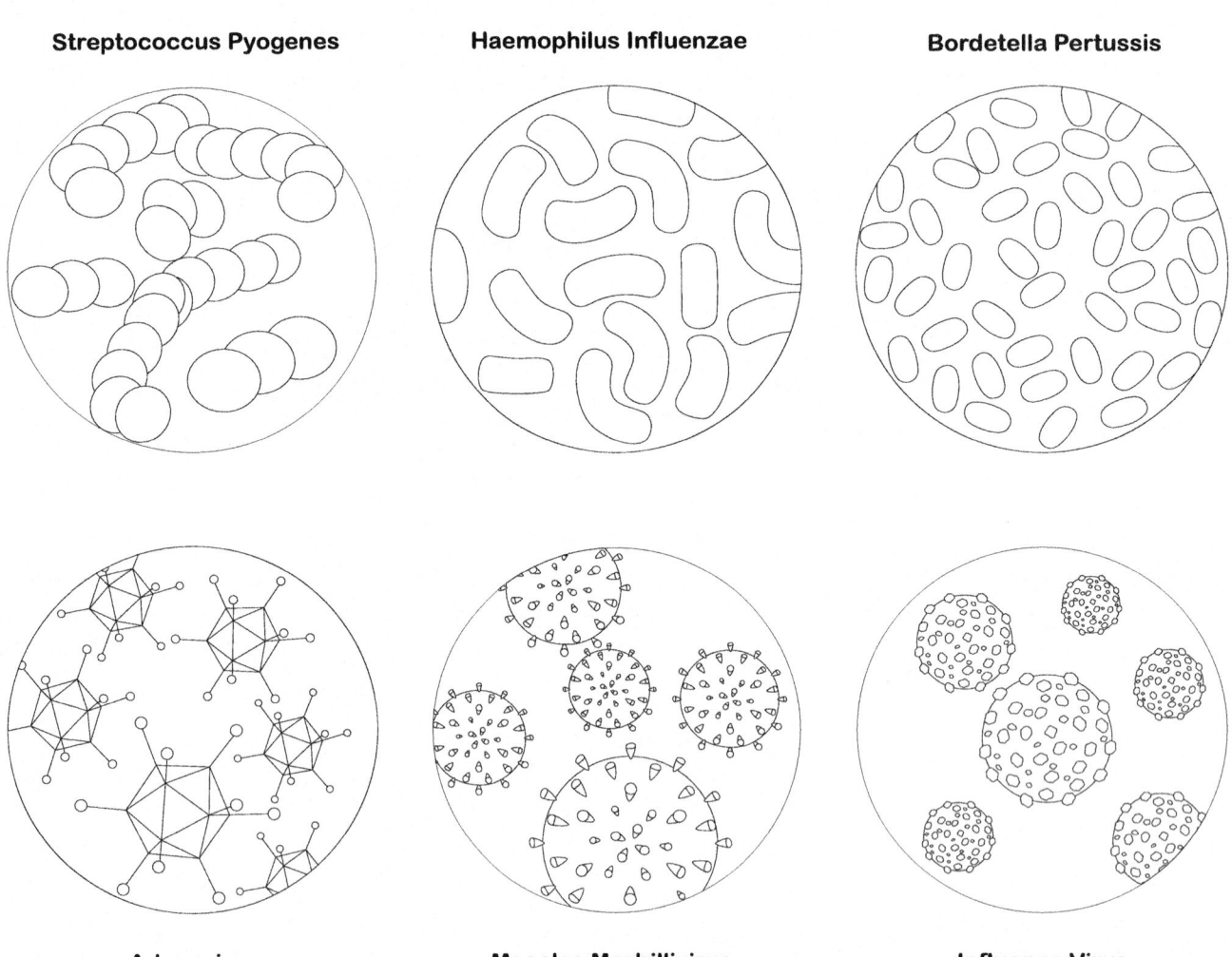

Sinusitis

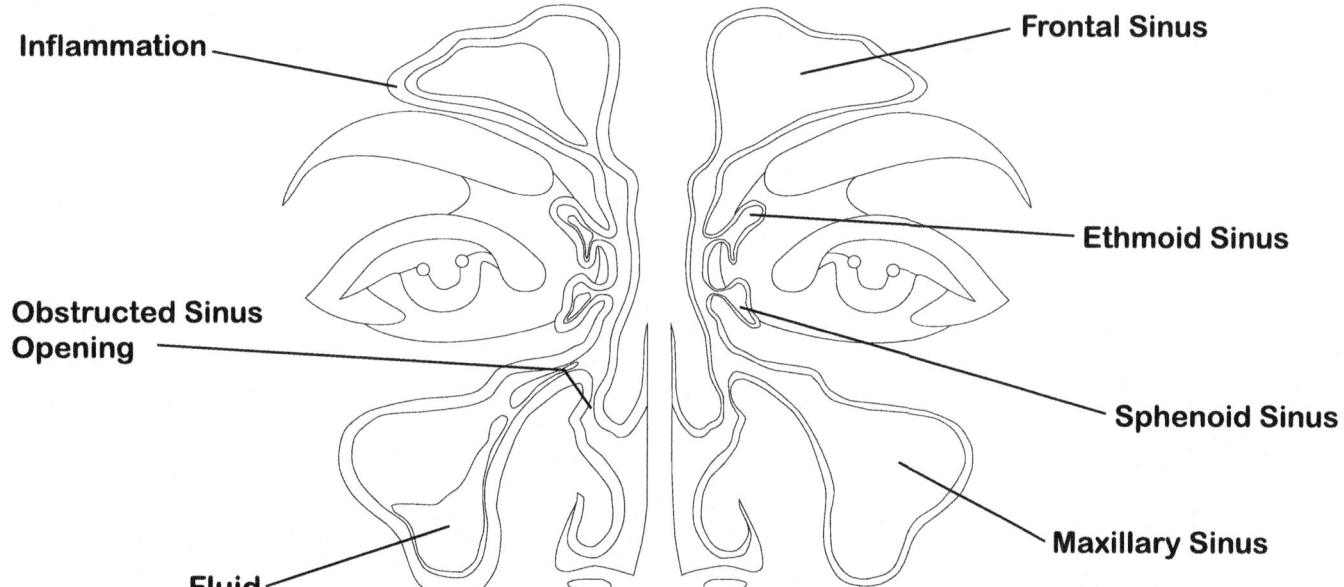

Tonsillitis

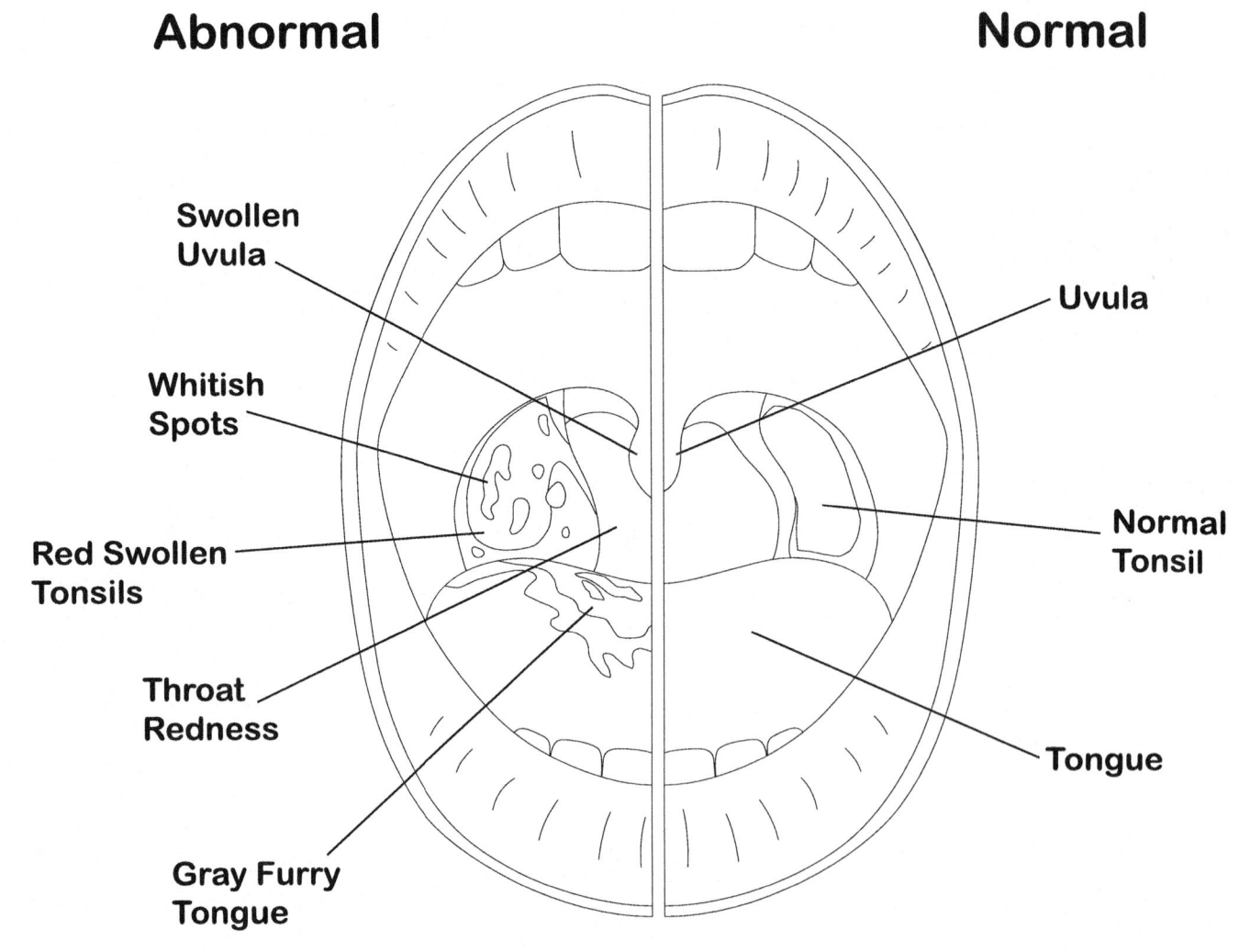

Laryngitis

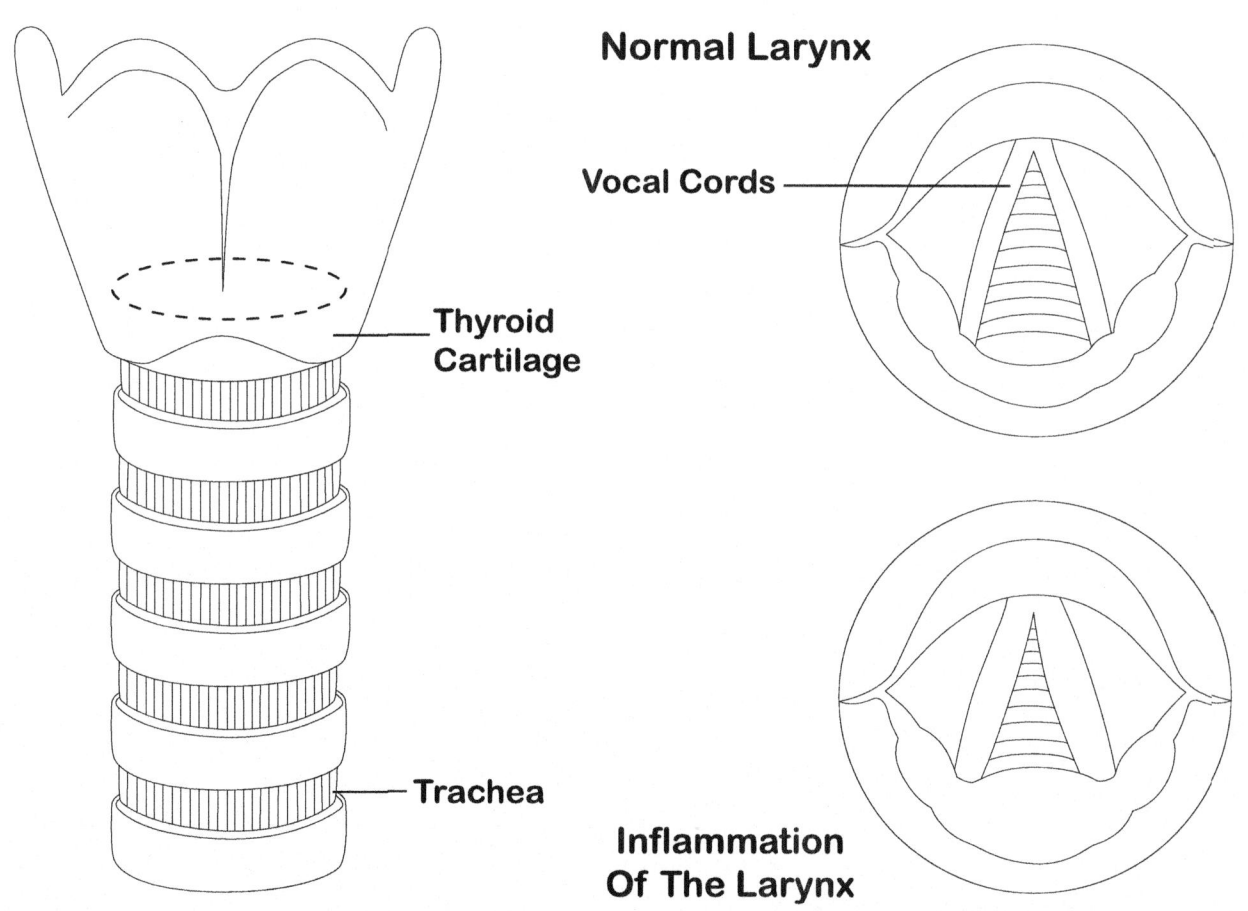

Epiglottis

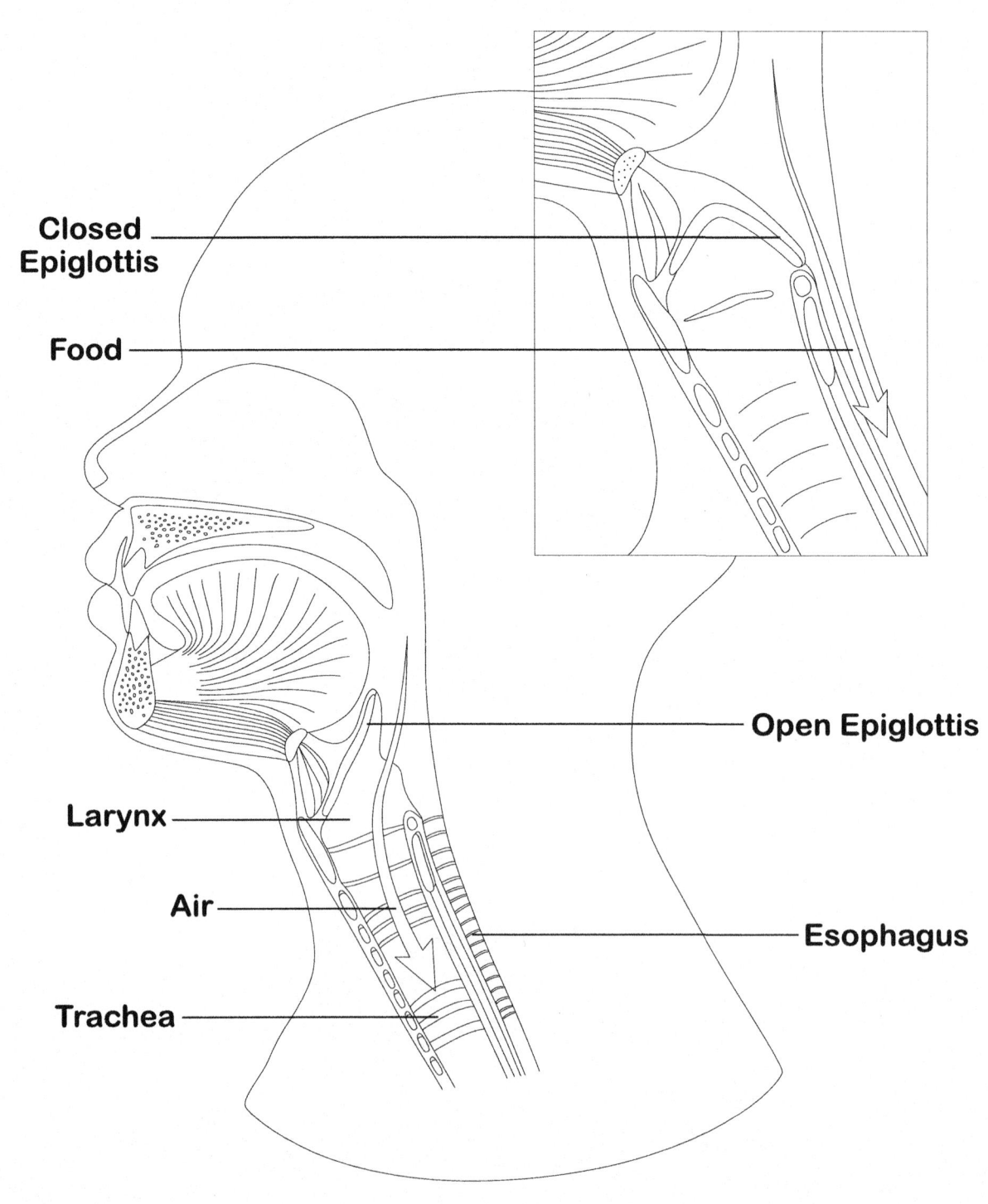

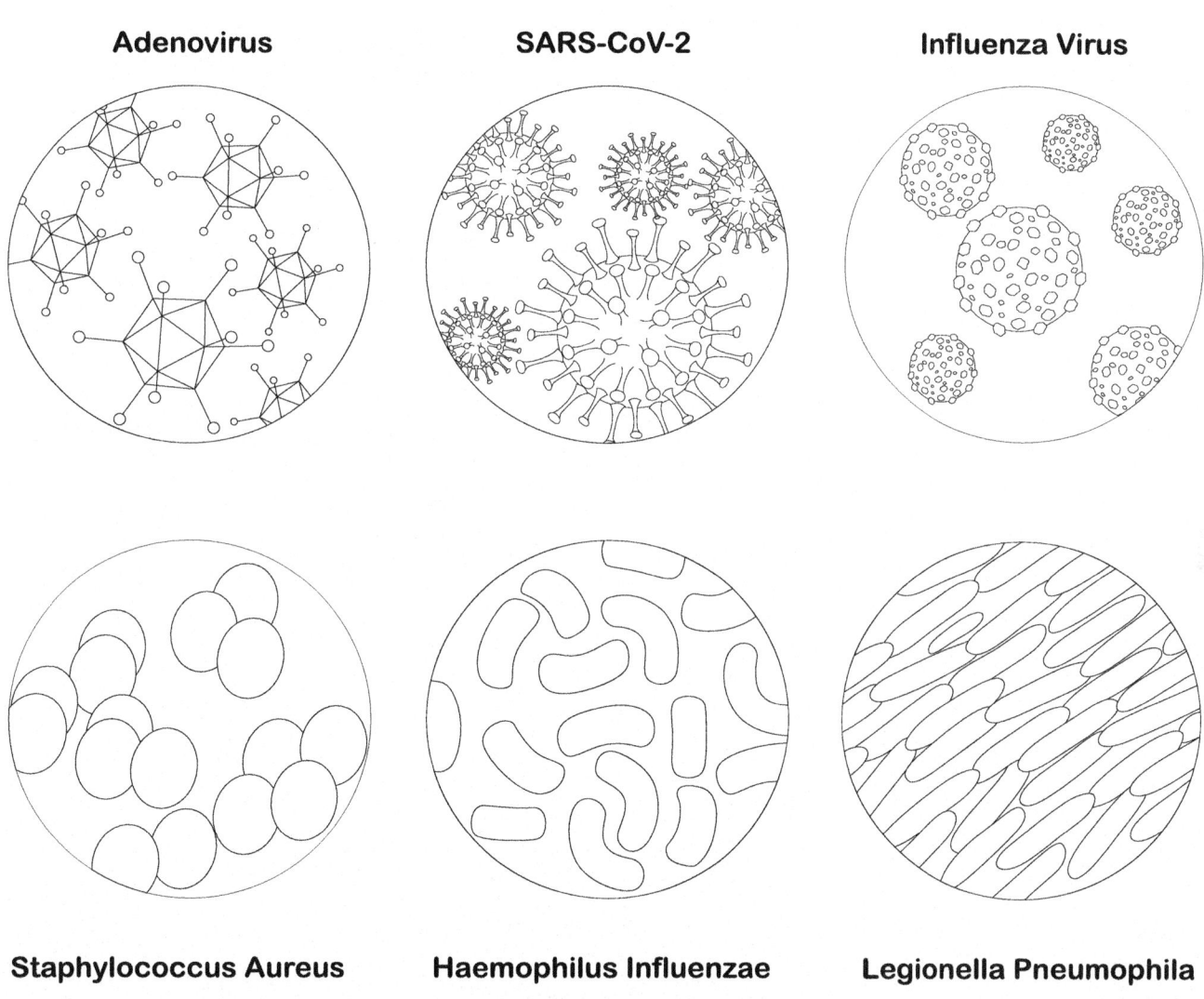

Pneumonia

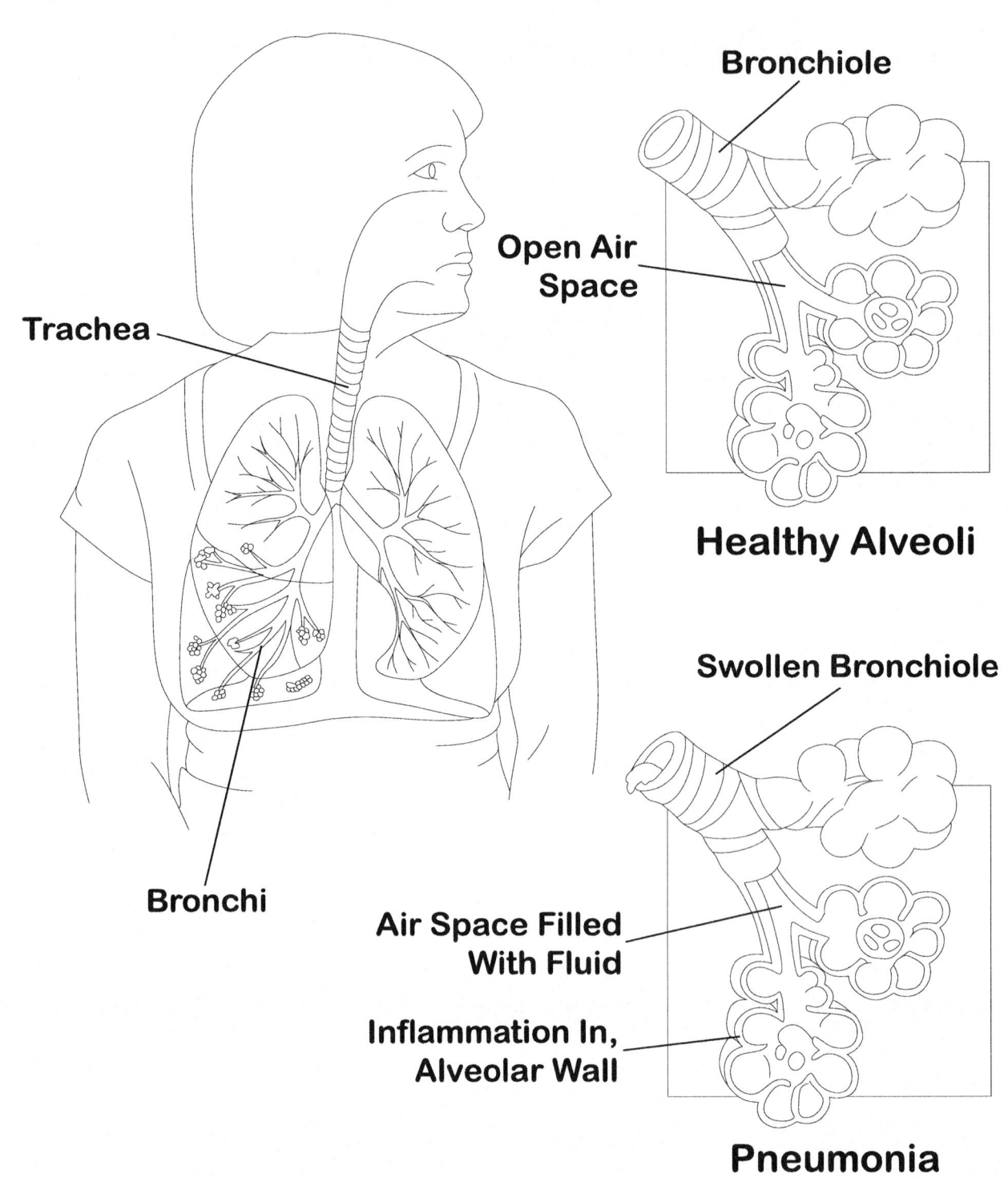

Bronchitis

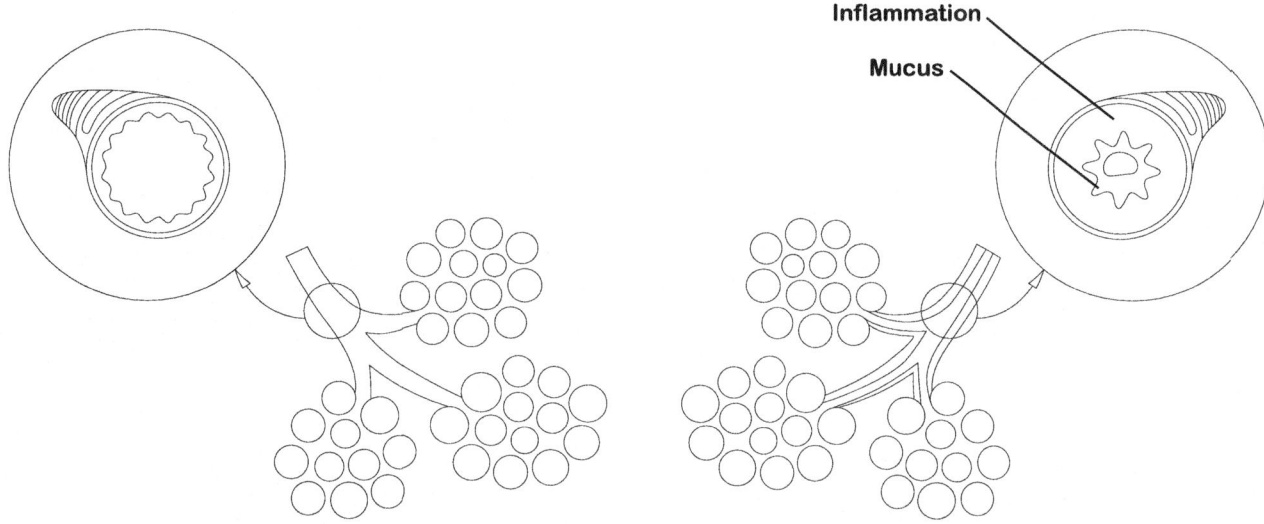

Healthy Lungs   Clogged Airways

Bronchiolitis

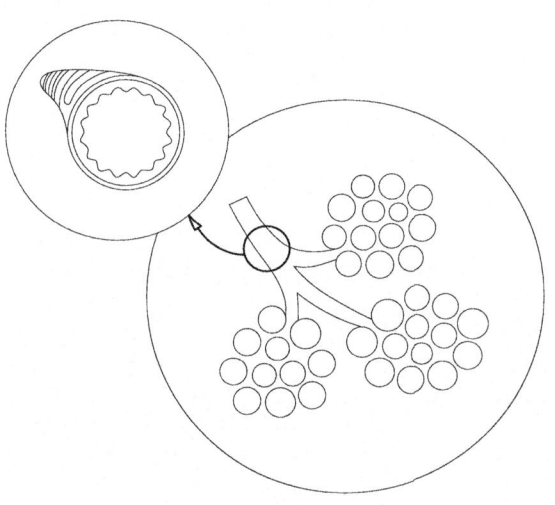 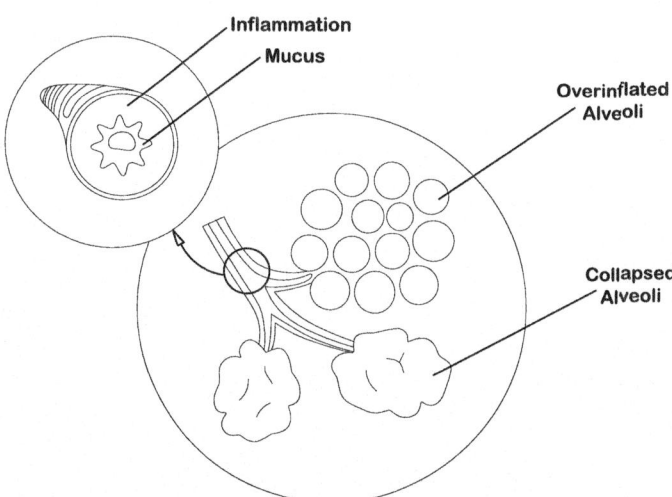

Healthy Lungs   Clogged Airways

Tuberculosis

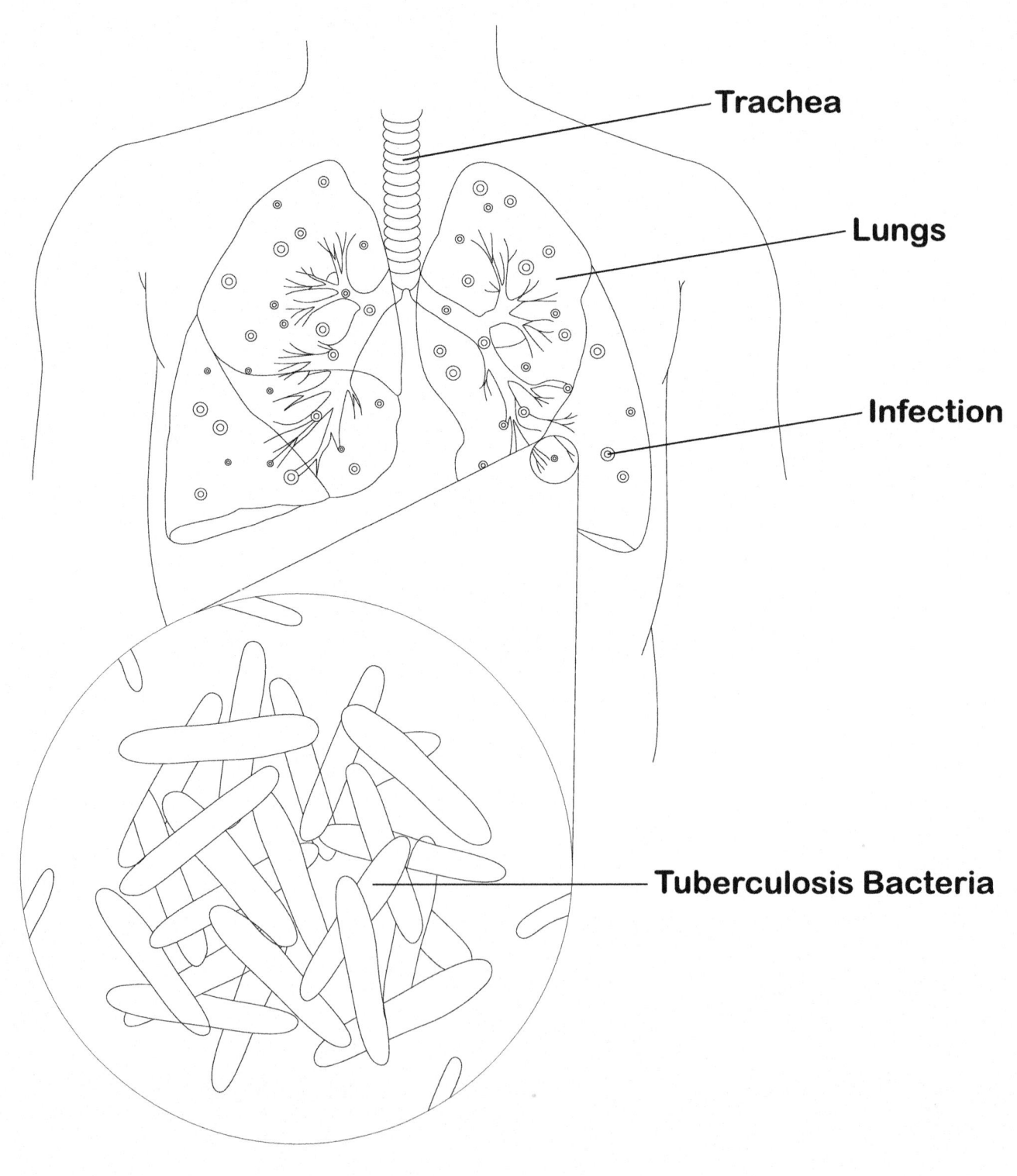

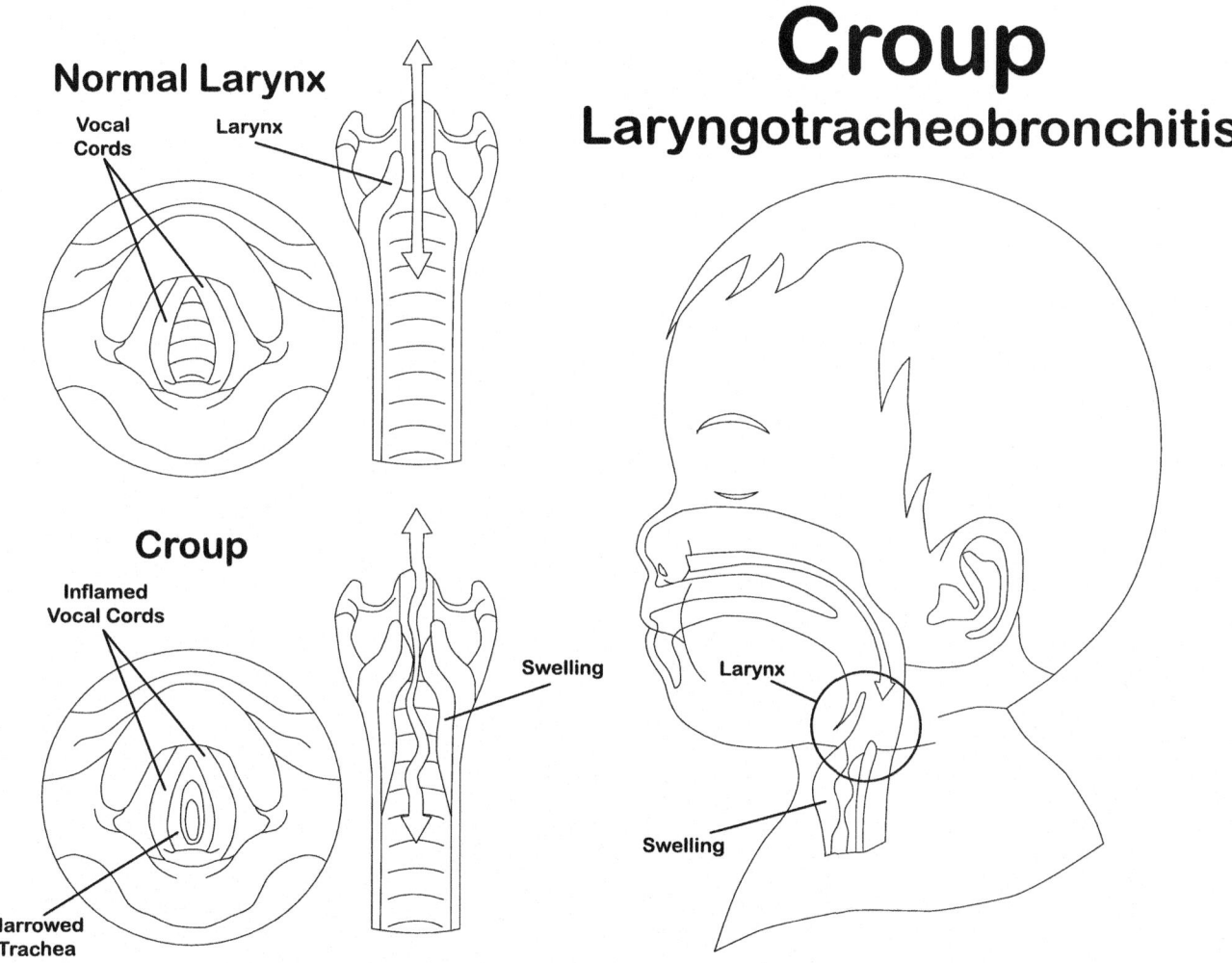

Asthma

Normal

- Relaxed Smooth Muscles
- Alveoli

Asthmatic

- Tightened Smooth Muscles
- Mucus

Chronic Obstructive Pulmonary Disease (COPD)

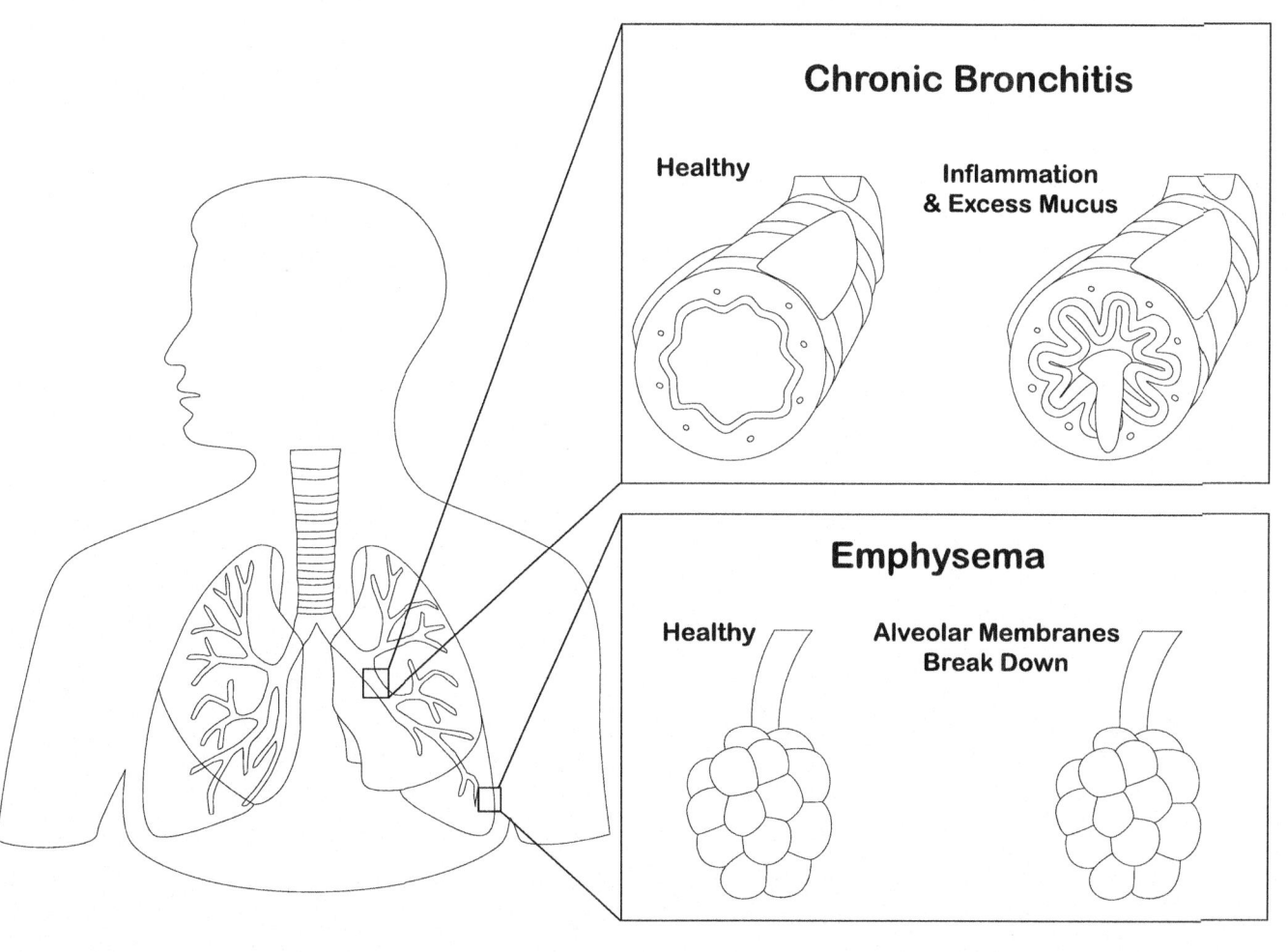

Obstructive Sleep Apnea (OSA)

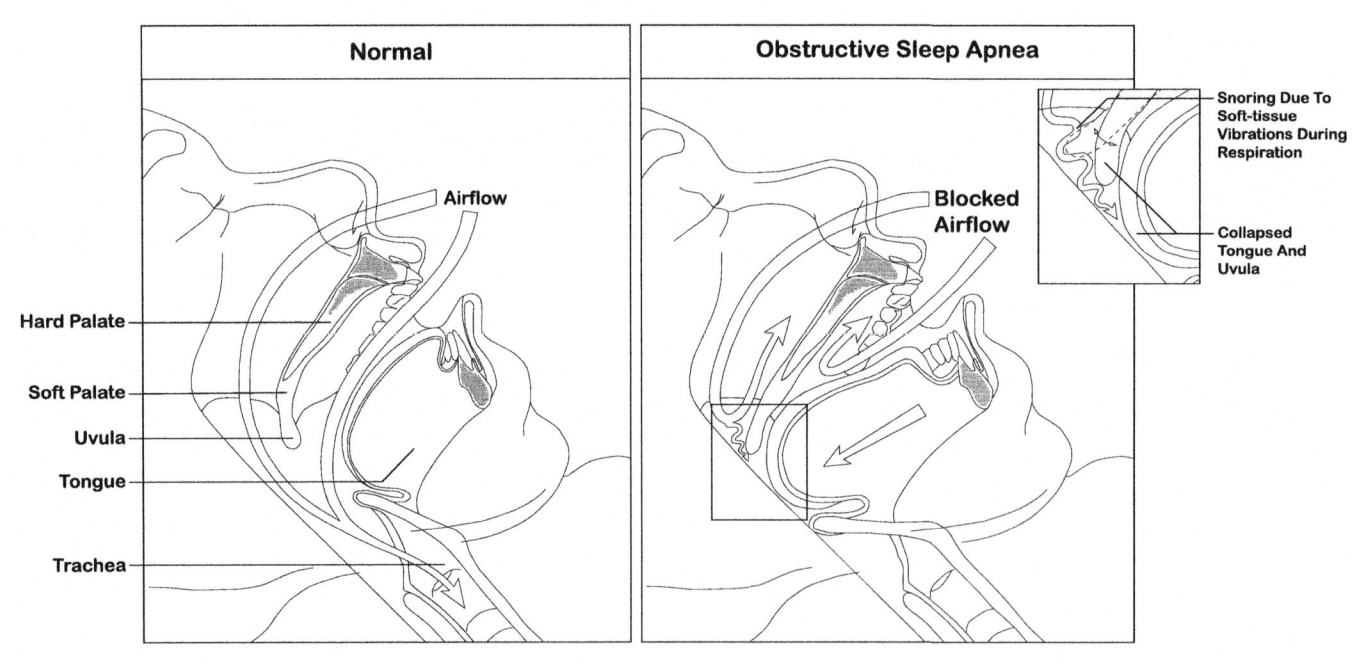

Cystic Fibrosis

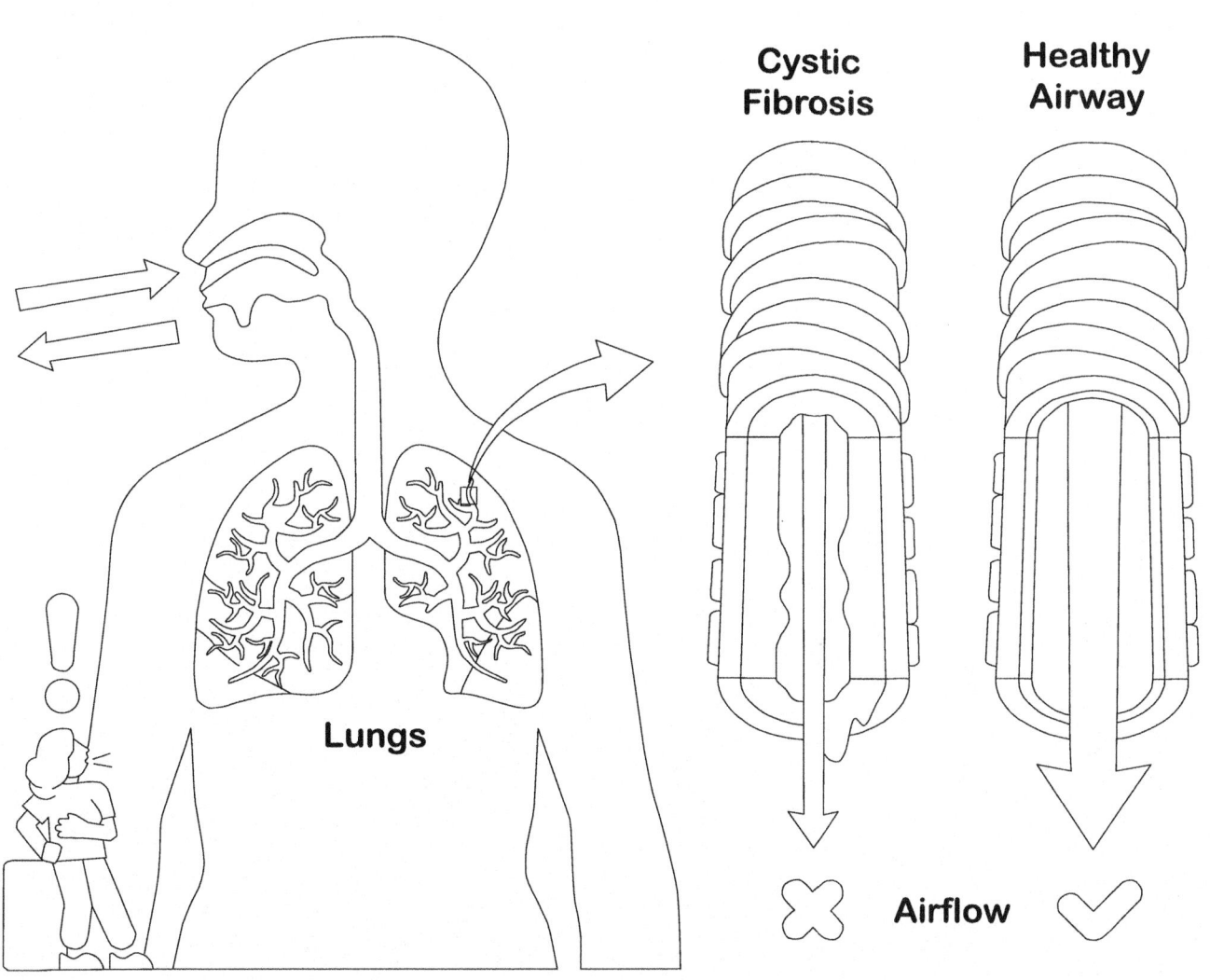

Lung Cancer

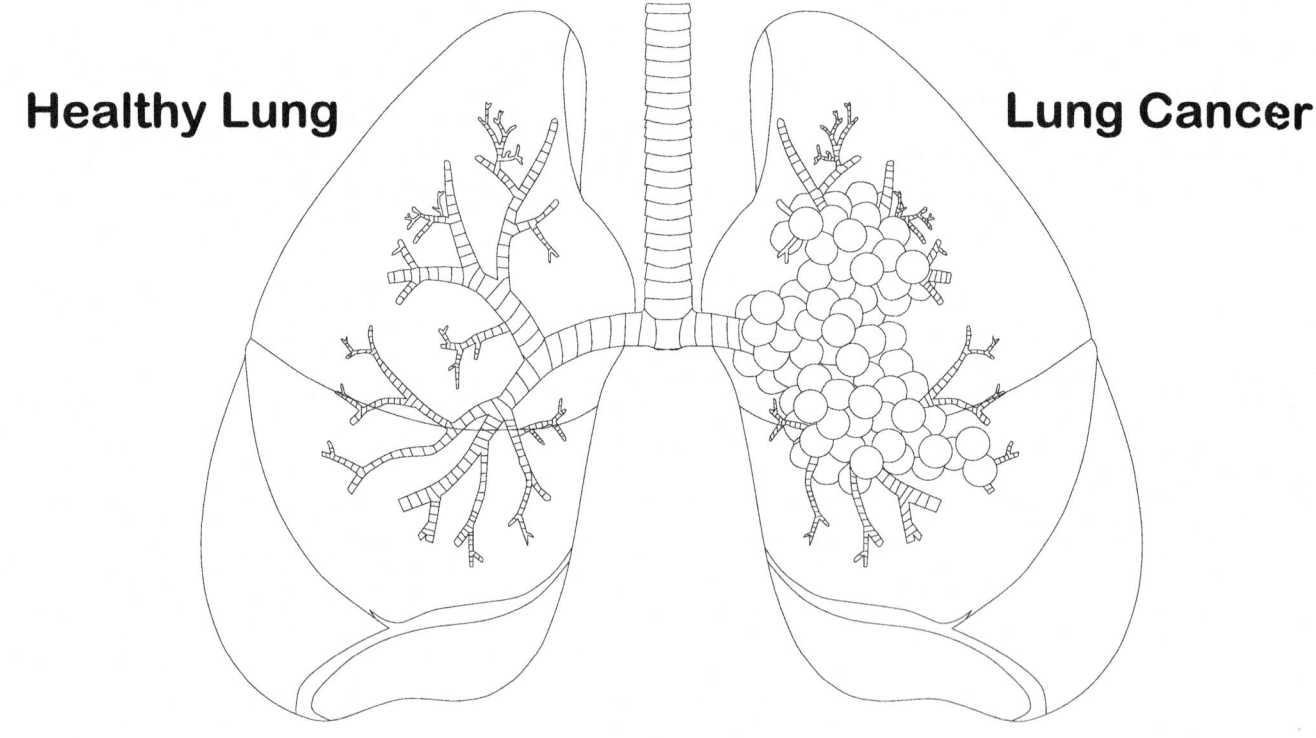

Healthy LungLung Cancer

Pulmonary Fibrosis

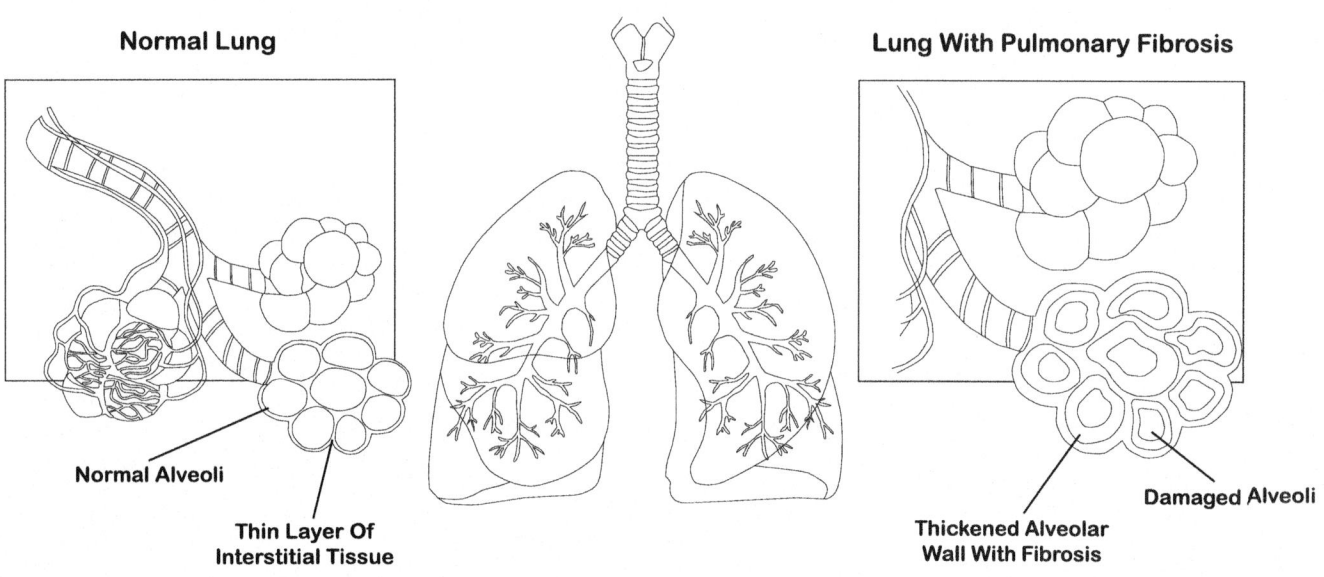

Sepsis

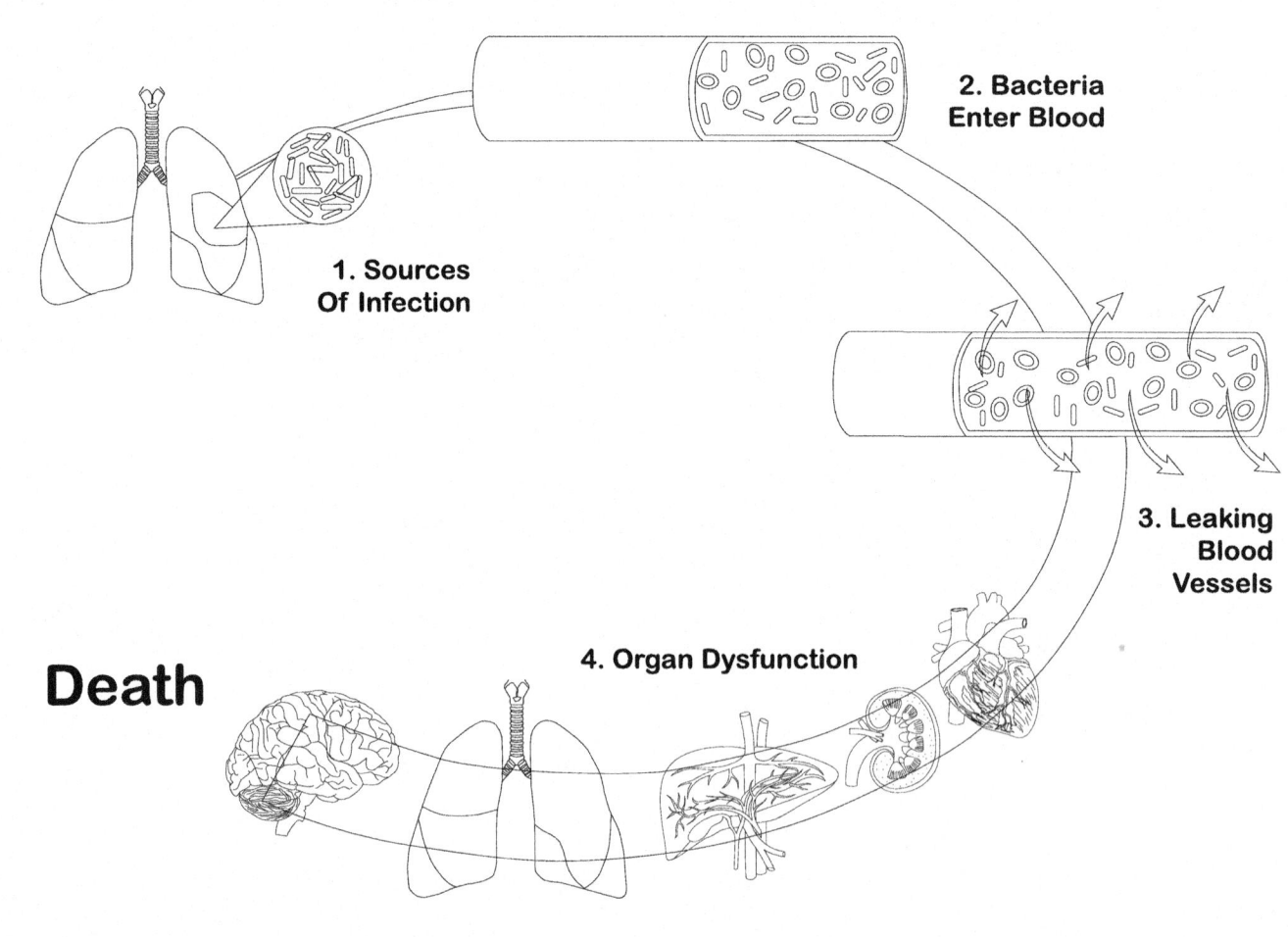

Bacteremia

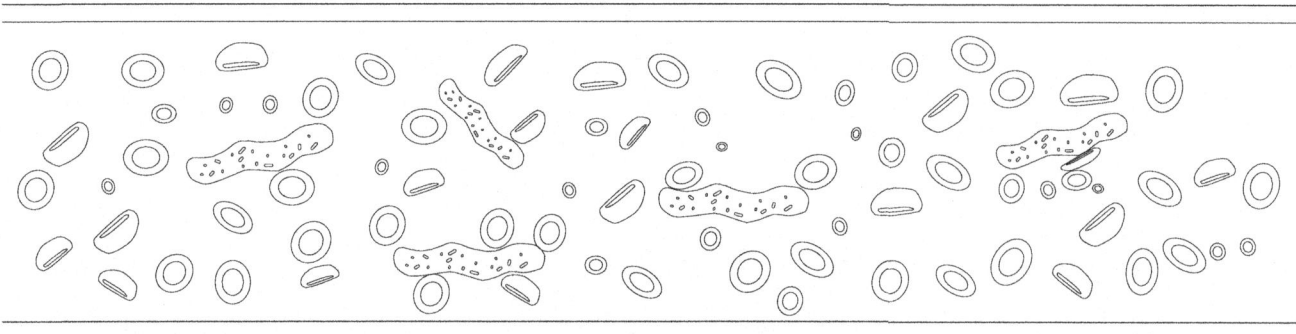

Bacteria In The Blood

Endocarditis

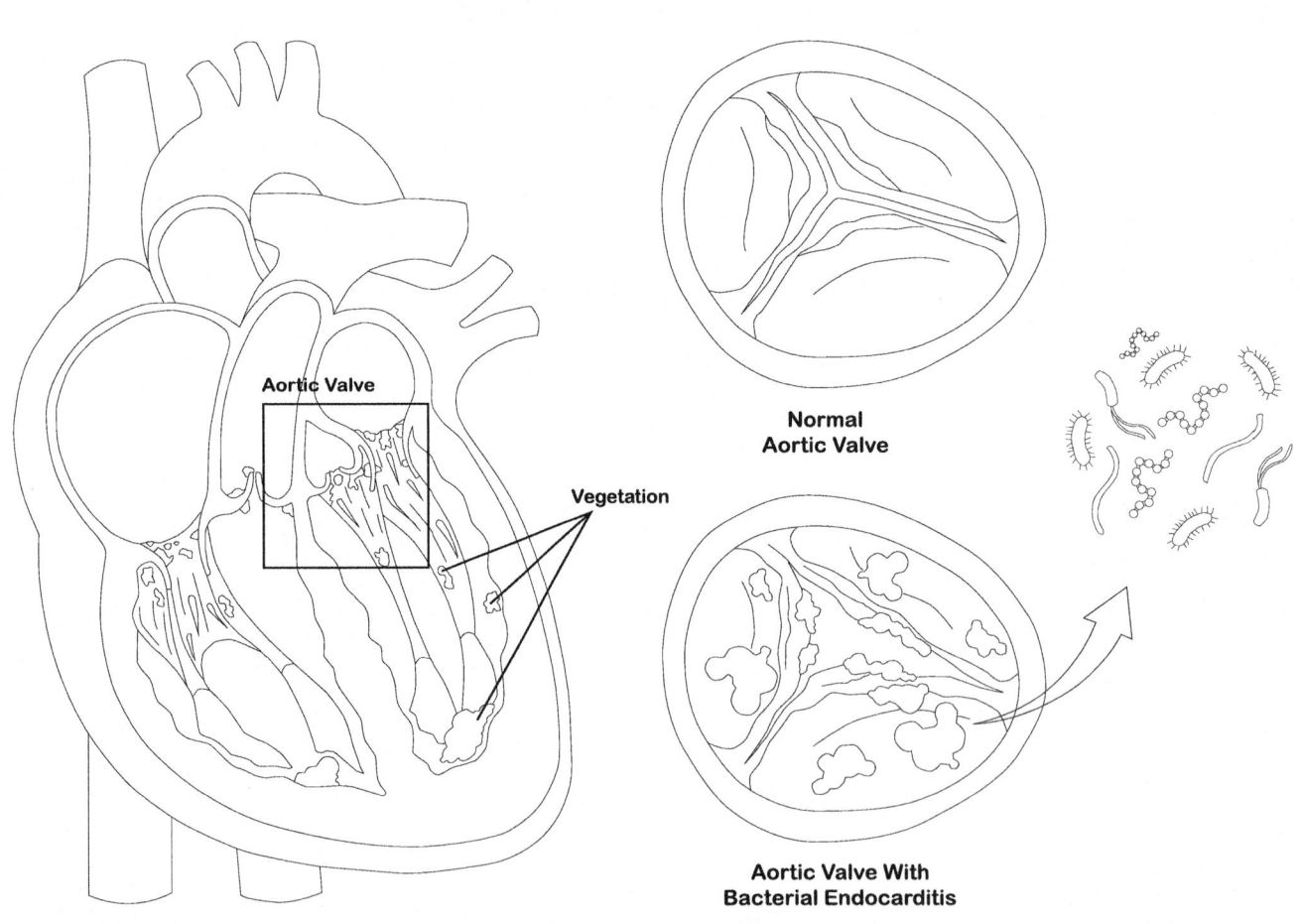

Pericarditis
Inflammation Of The Pericardium

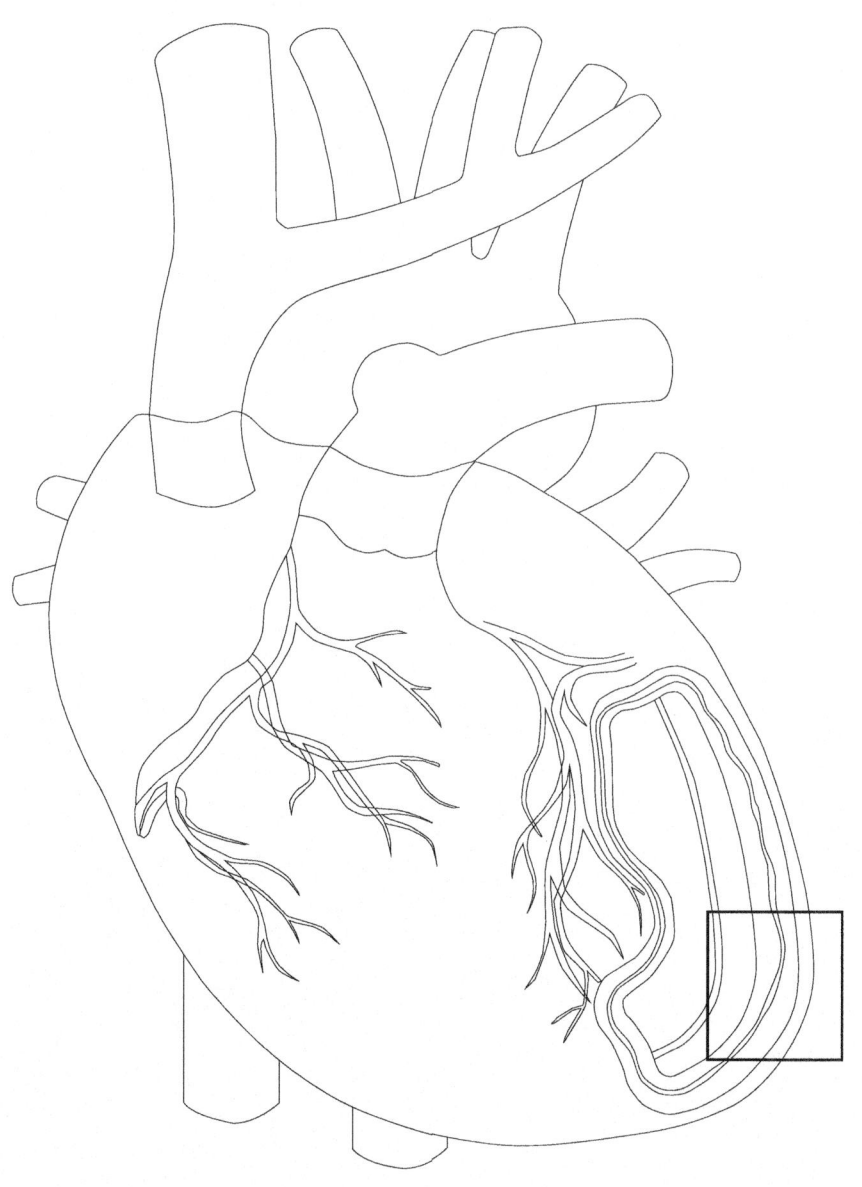

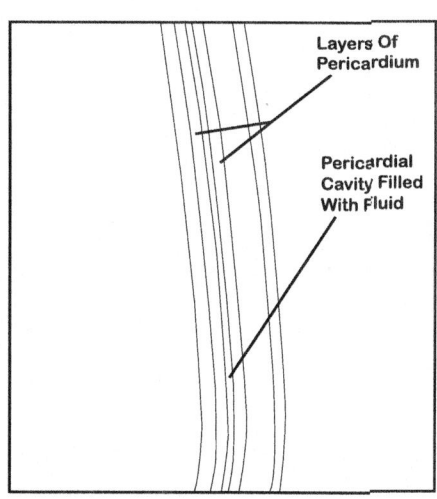

Normal Pericardium

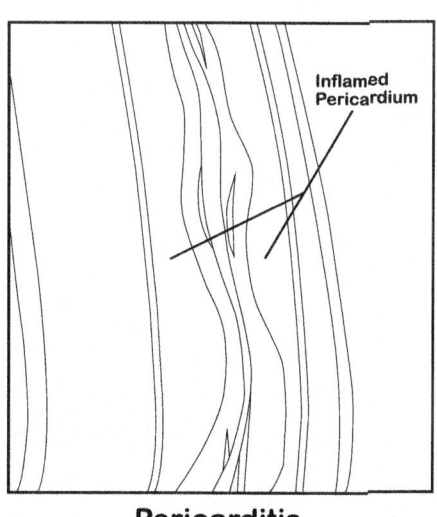

Pericarditis

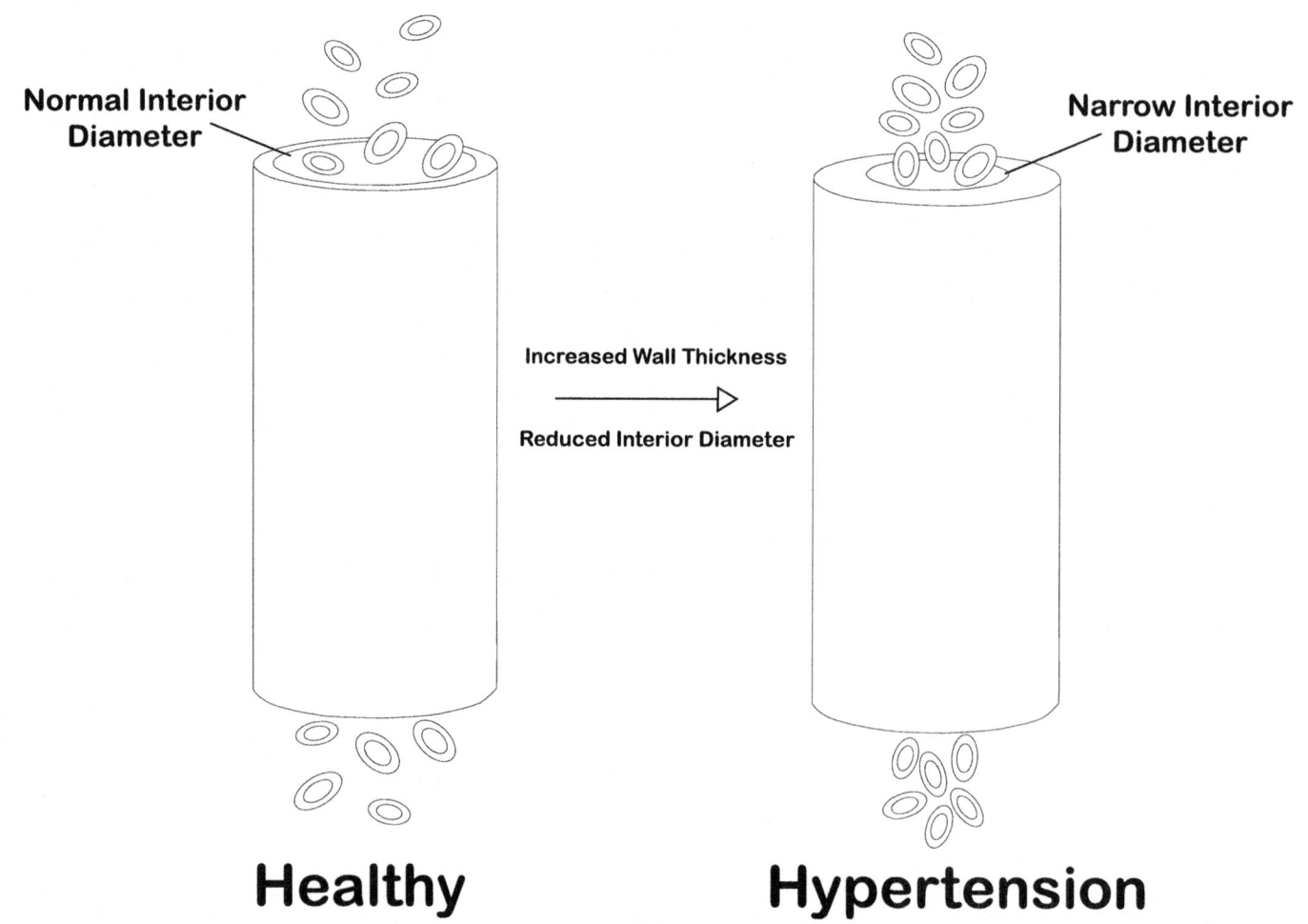

Coronary Artery Disease

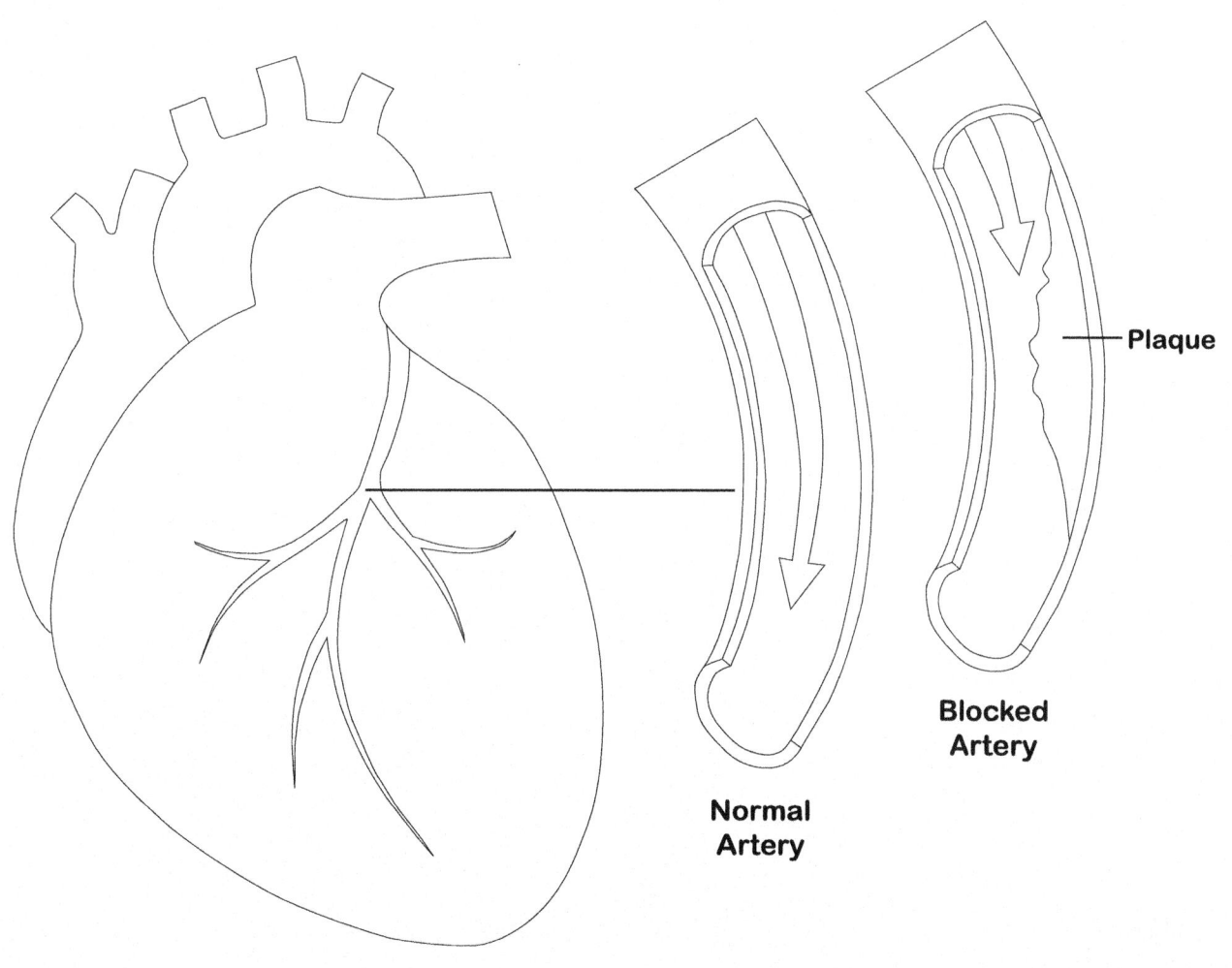

Myocardial Infarction

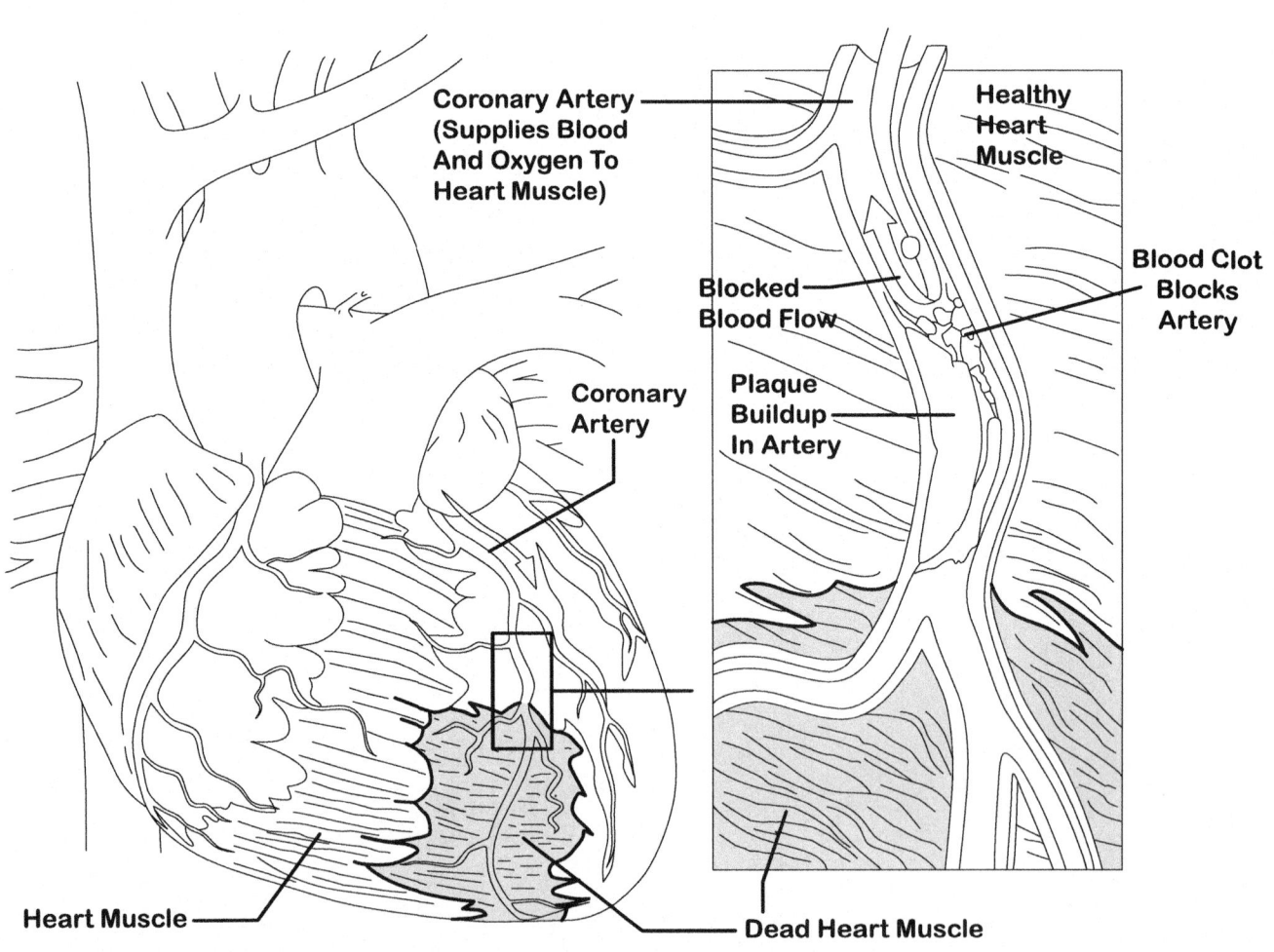

Heart Failure

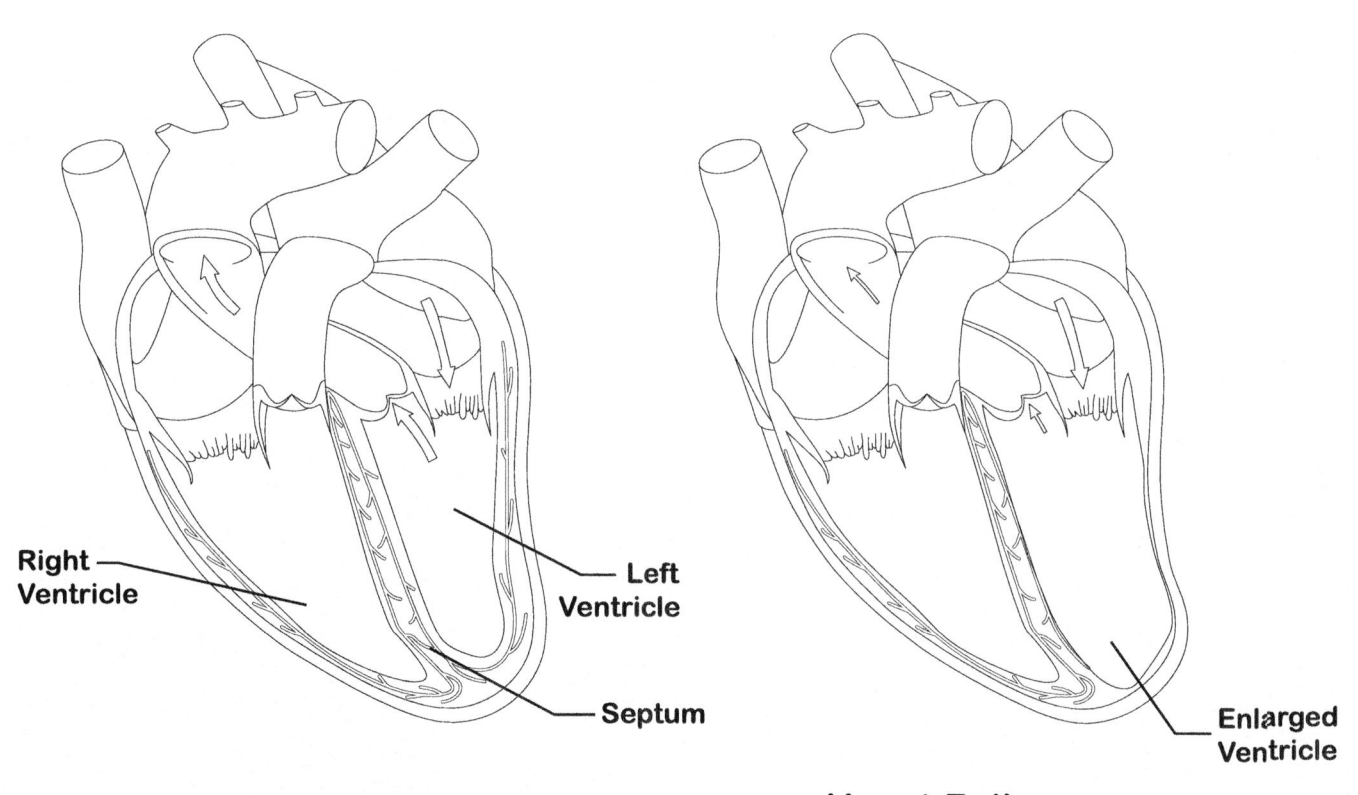

Normal Heart

Heart Failure

Cardiac Arrhythmia

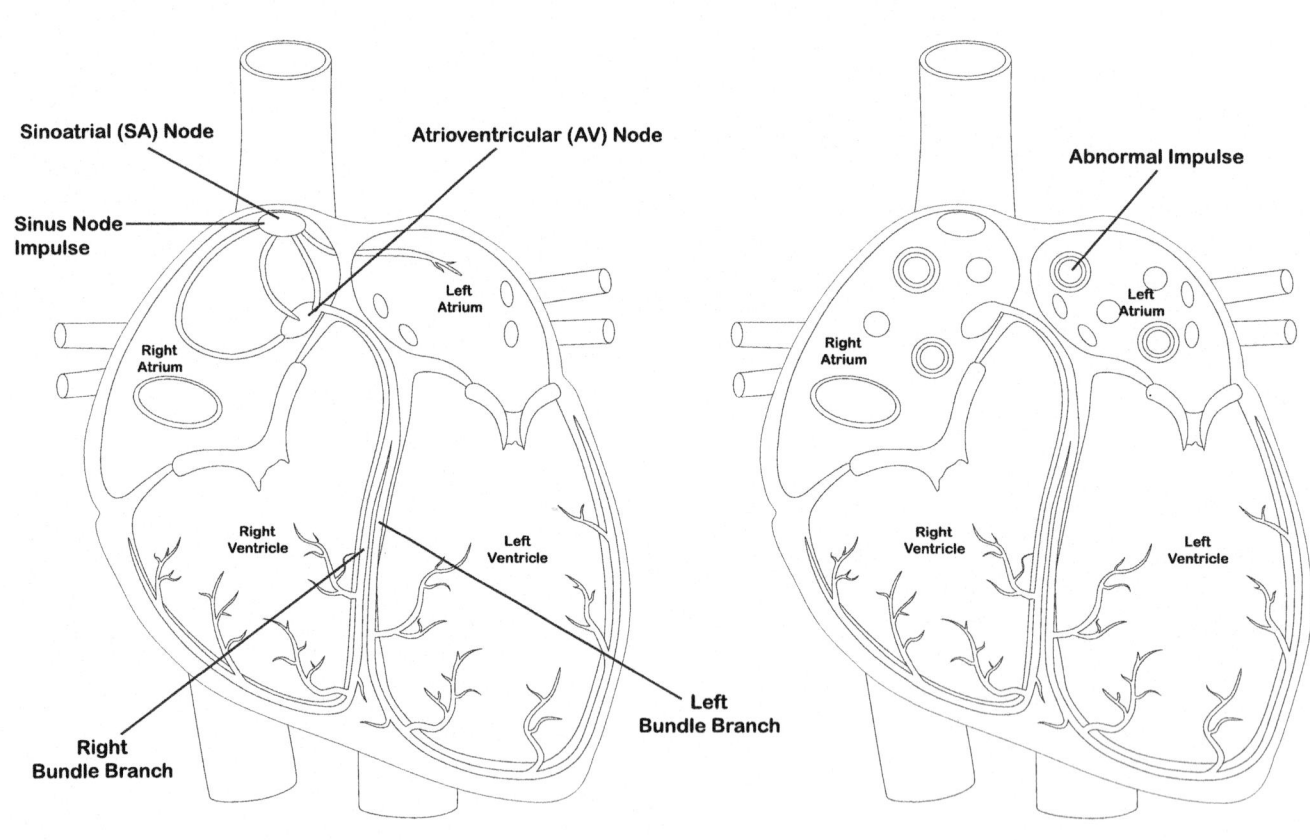

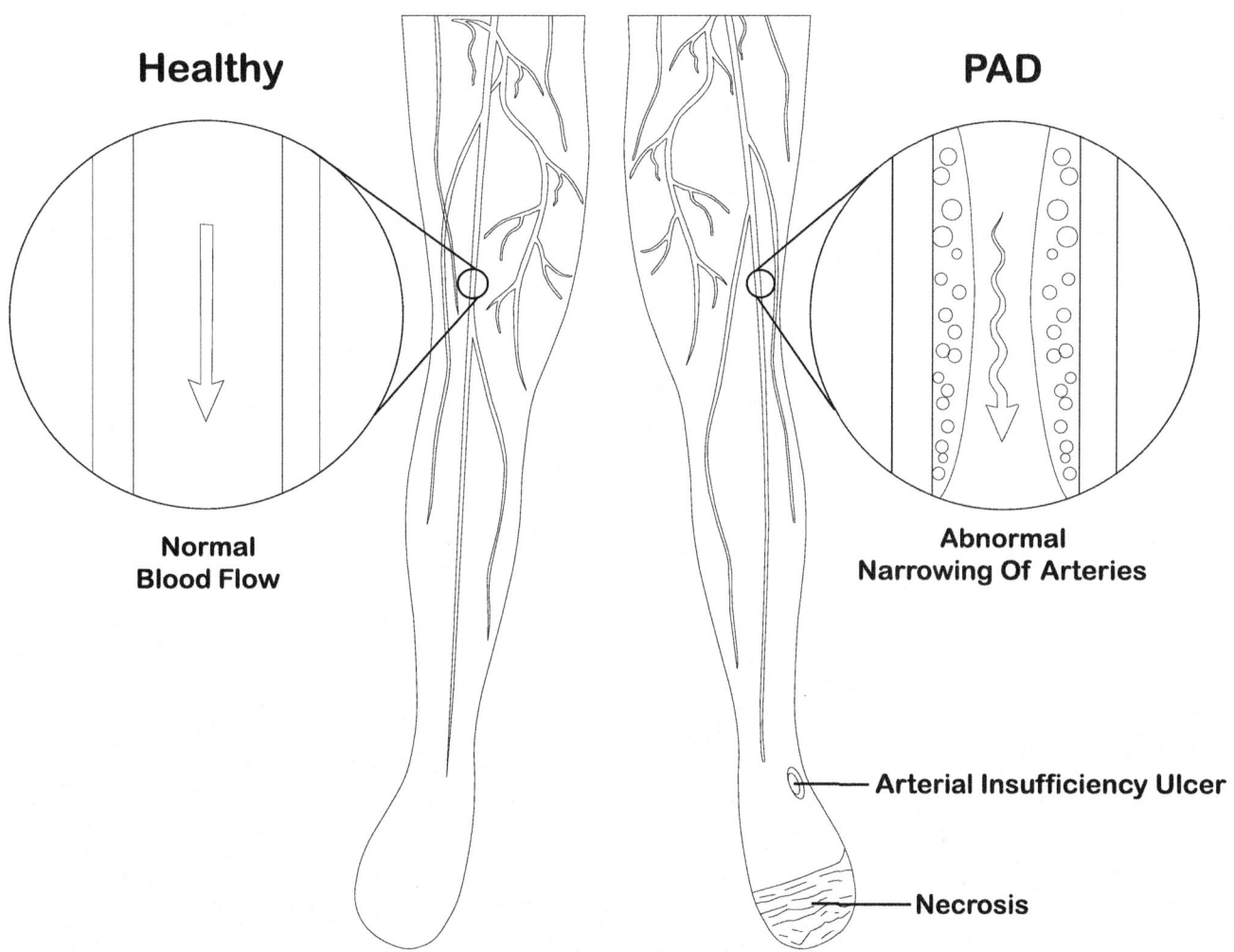

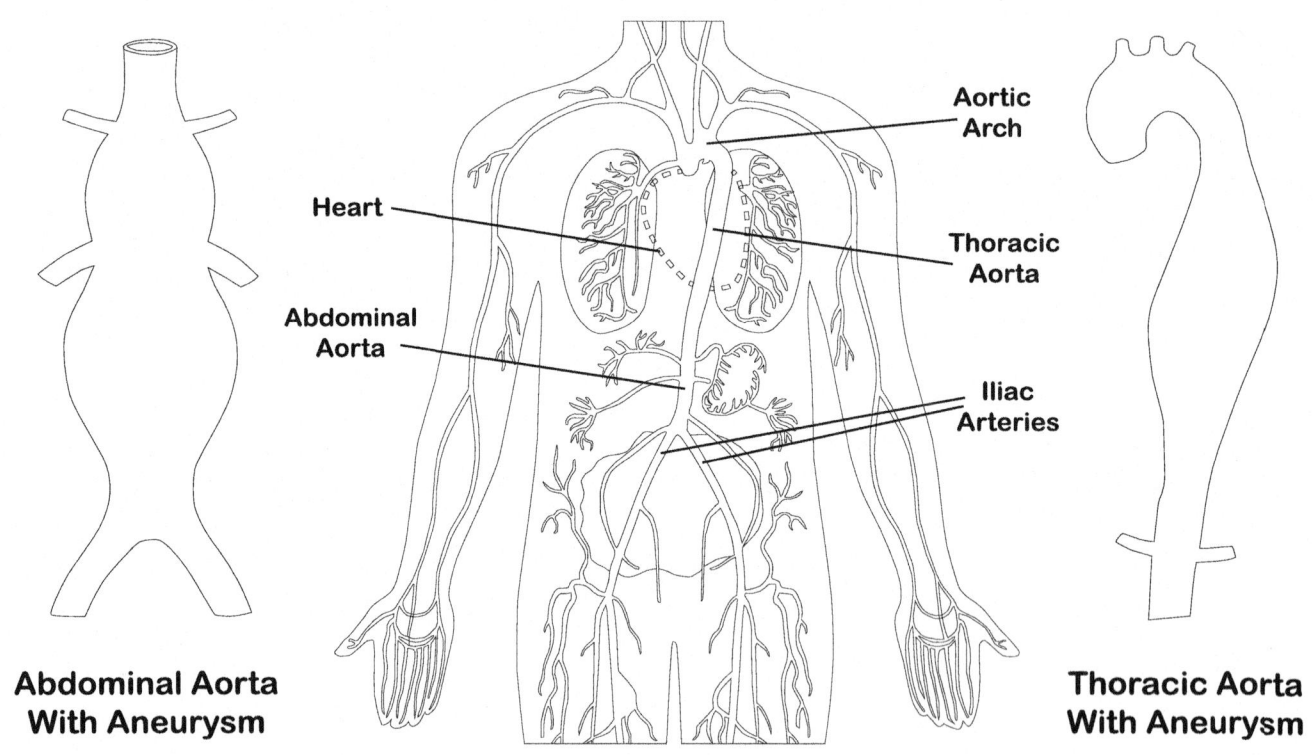

Deep Vein Thrombosis (DTV)

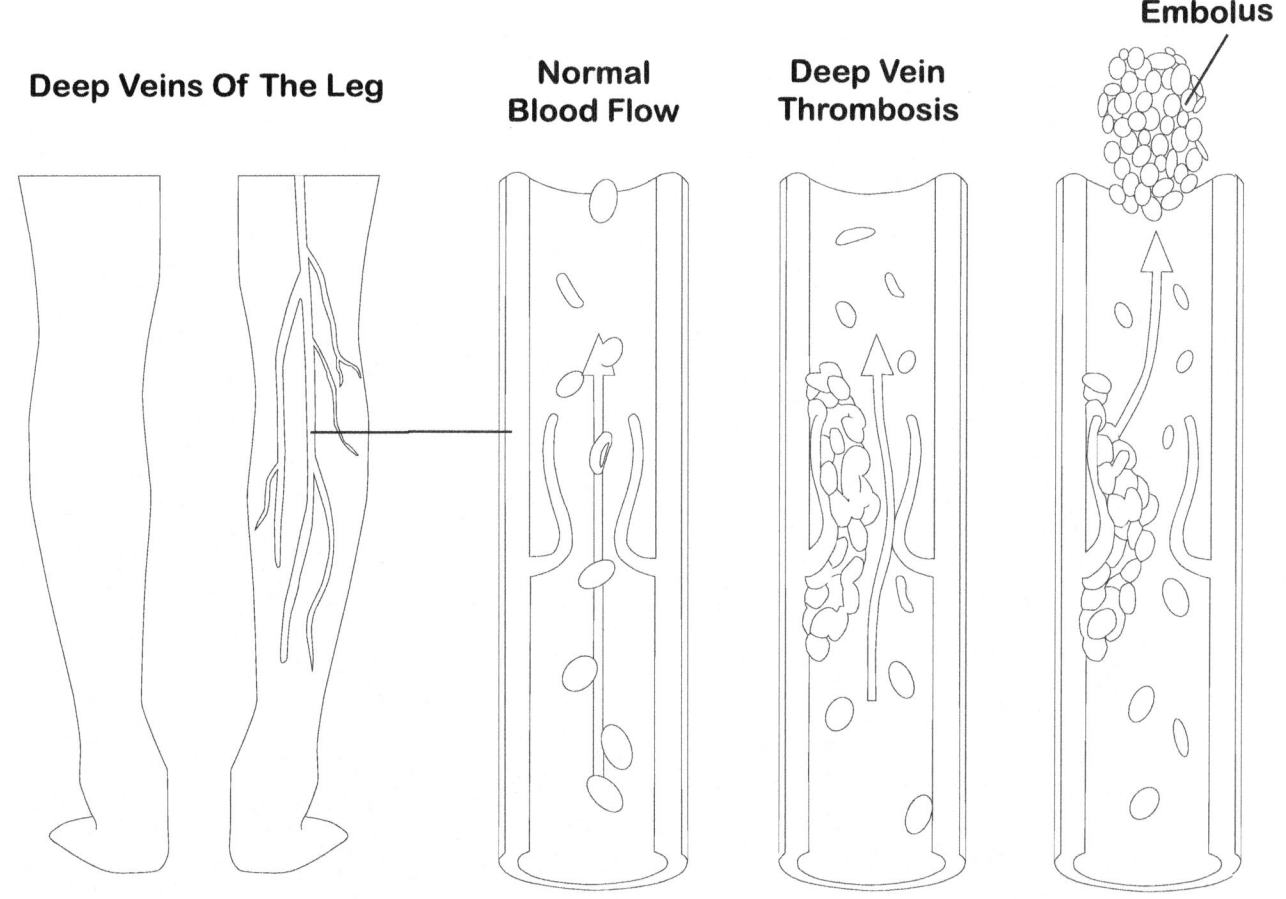

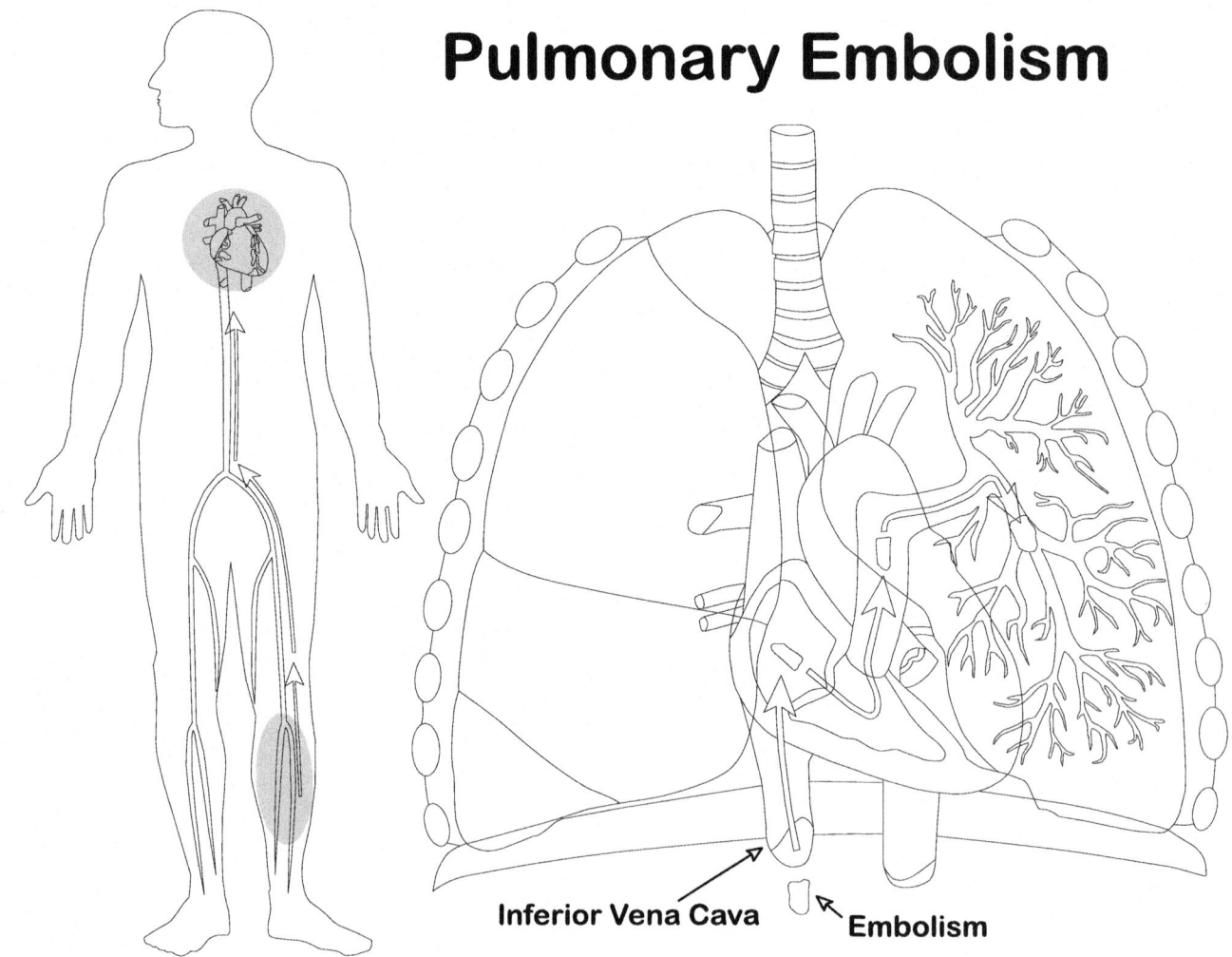

Cardiomyopathy

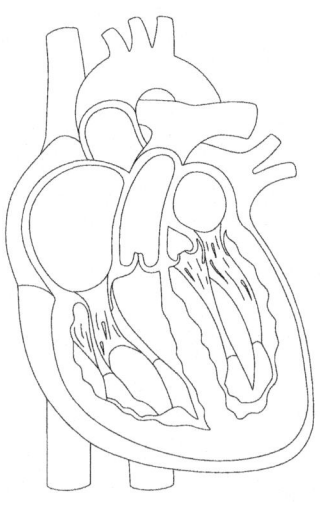

Normal Heart

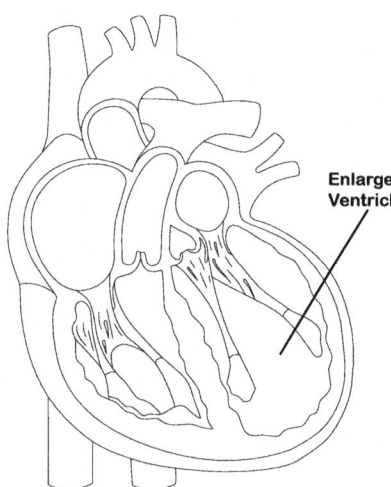

Dilated Cardiomyopathy

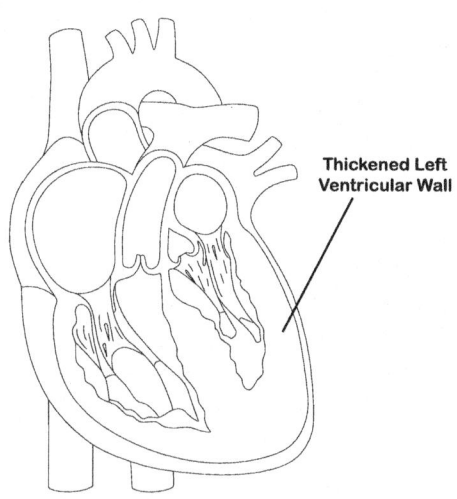

Hypertrophic Cardiomyopathy

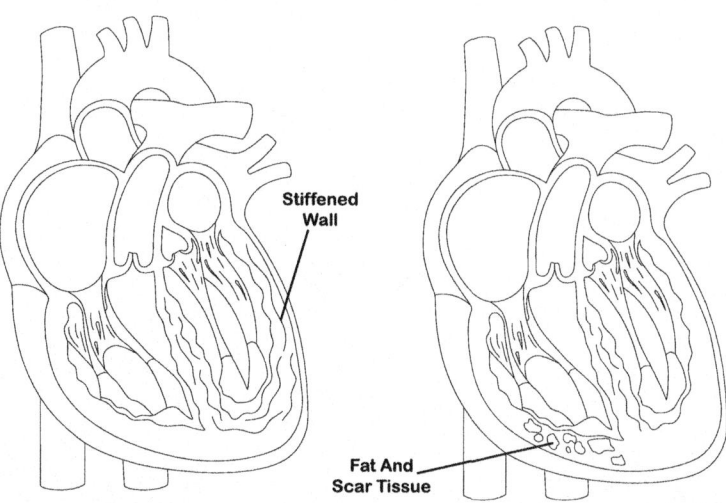

Restrictive Cardiomyopathy

Arrhythmogenic Cardiomyopathy

Heart Valve Disease

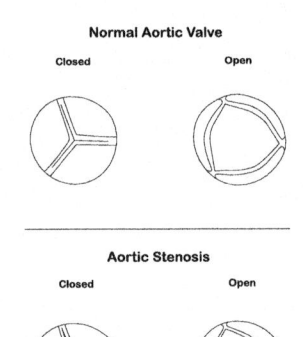
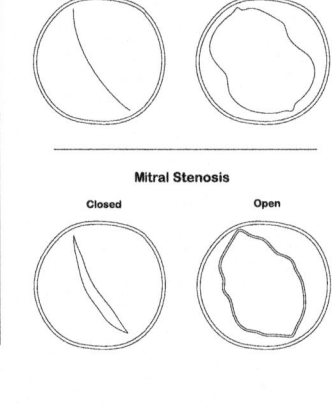
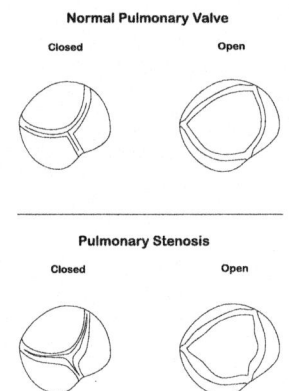
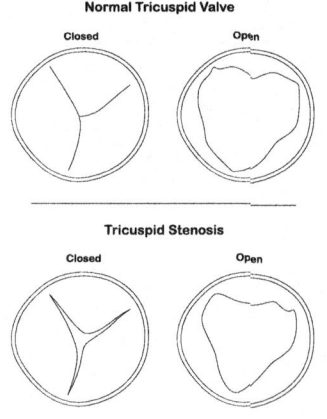

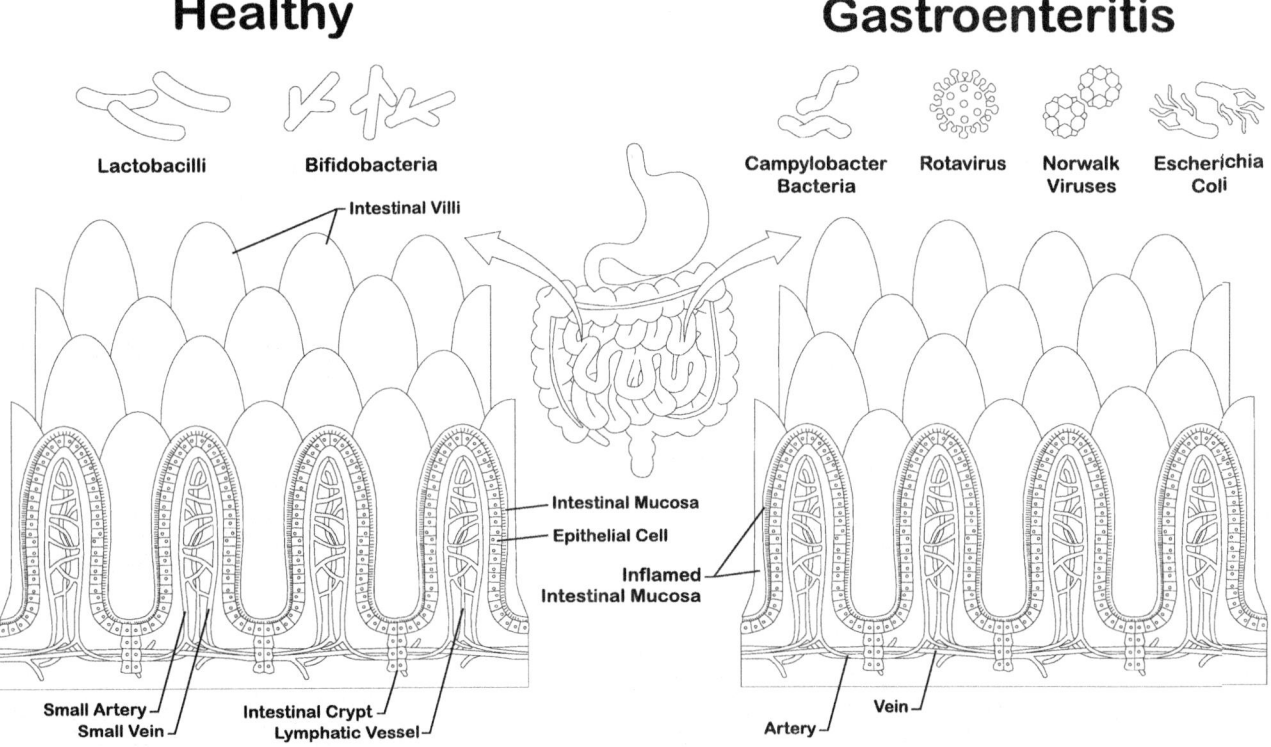

Peptic Ulcer Disease

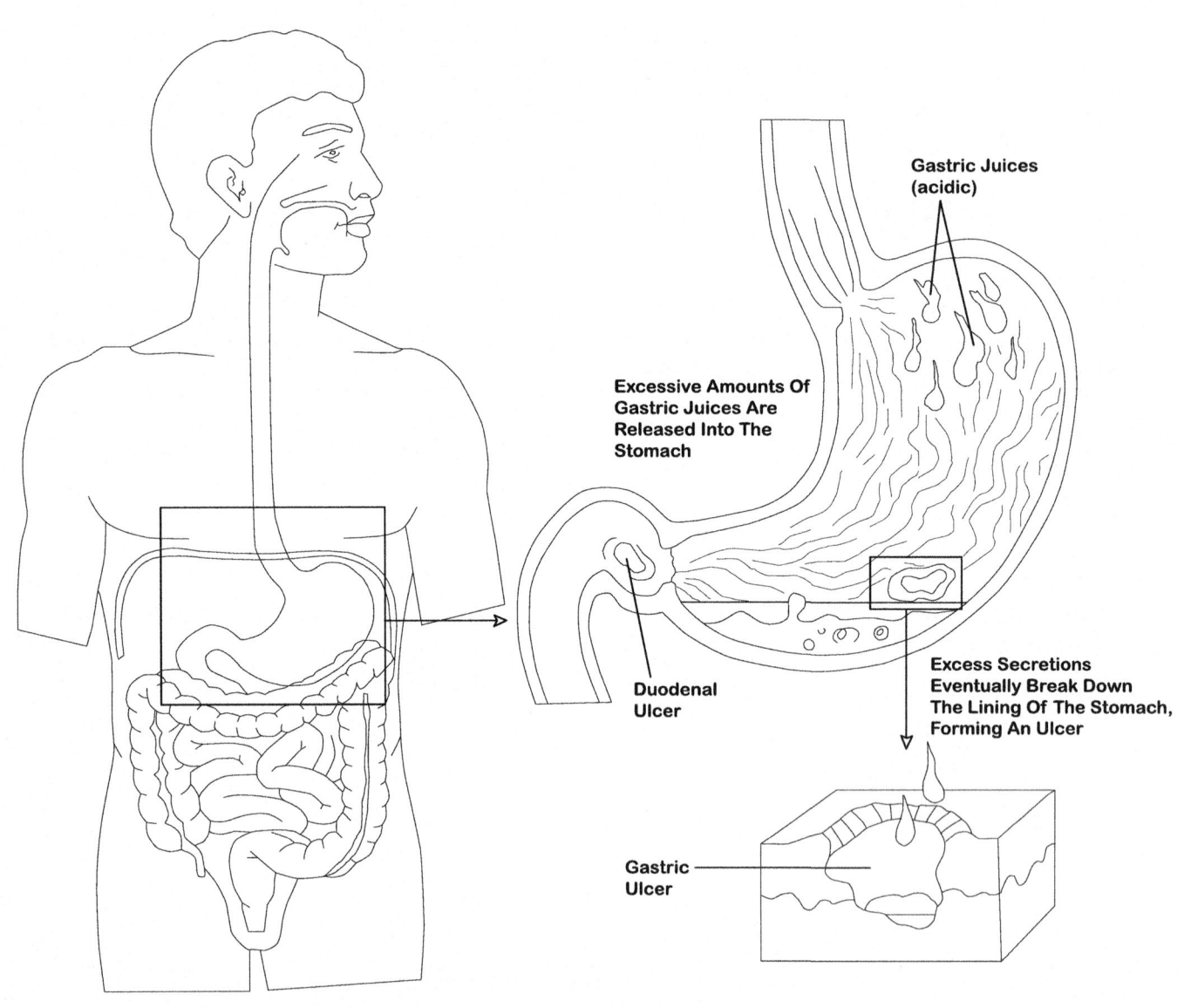

Gastroesophageal Reflux Disease

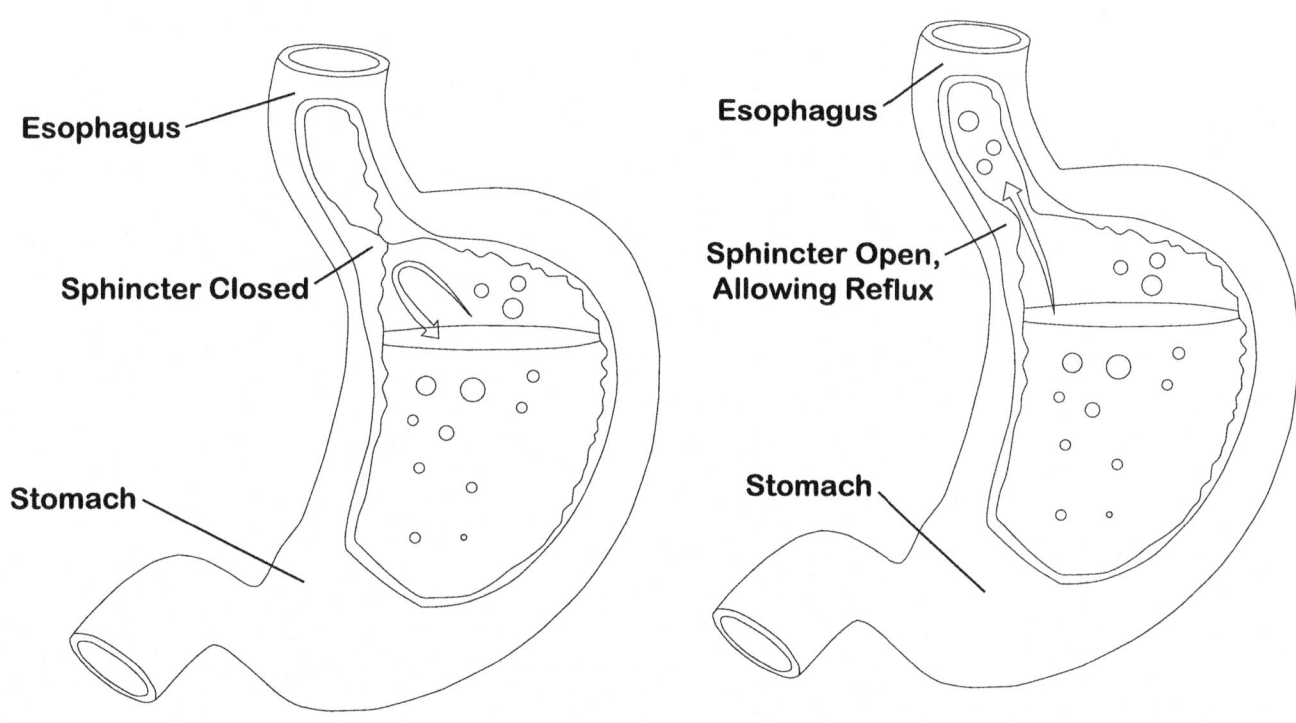

Healthy　　　　　　　　　　GERD

Gastritis

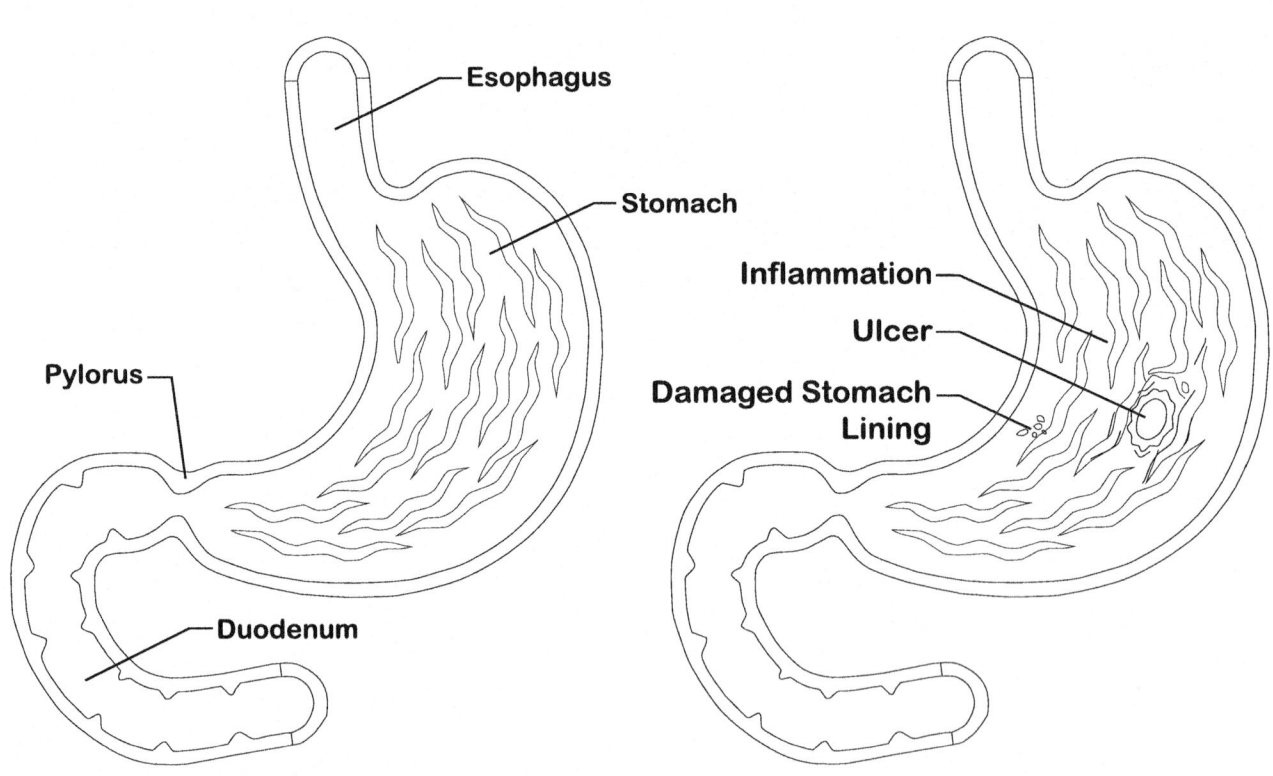

Ulcerative Colitis (Inflammatory Bowel Disease: IBD)

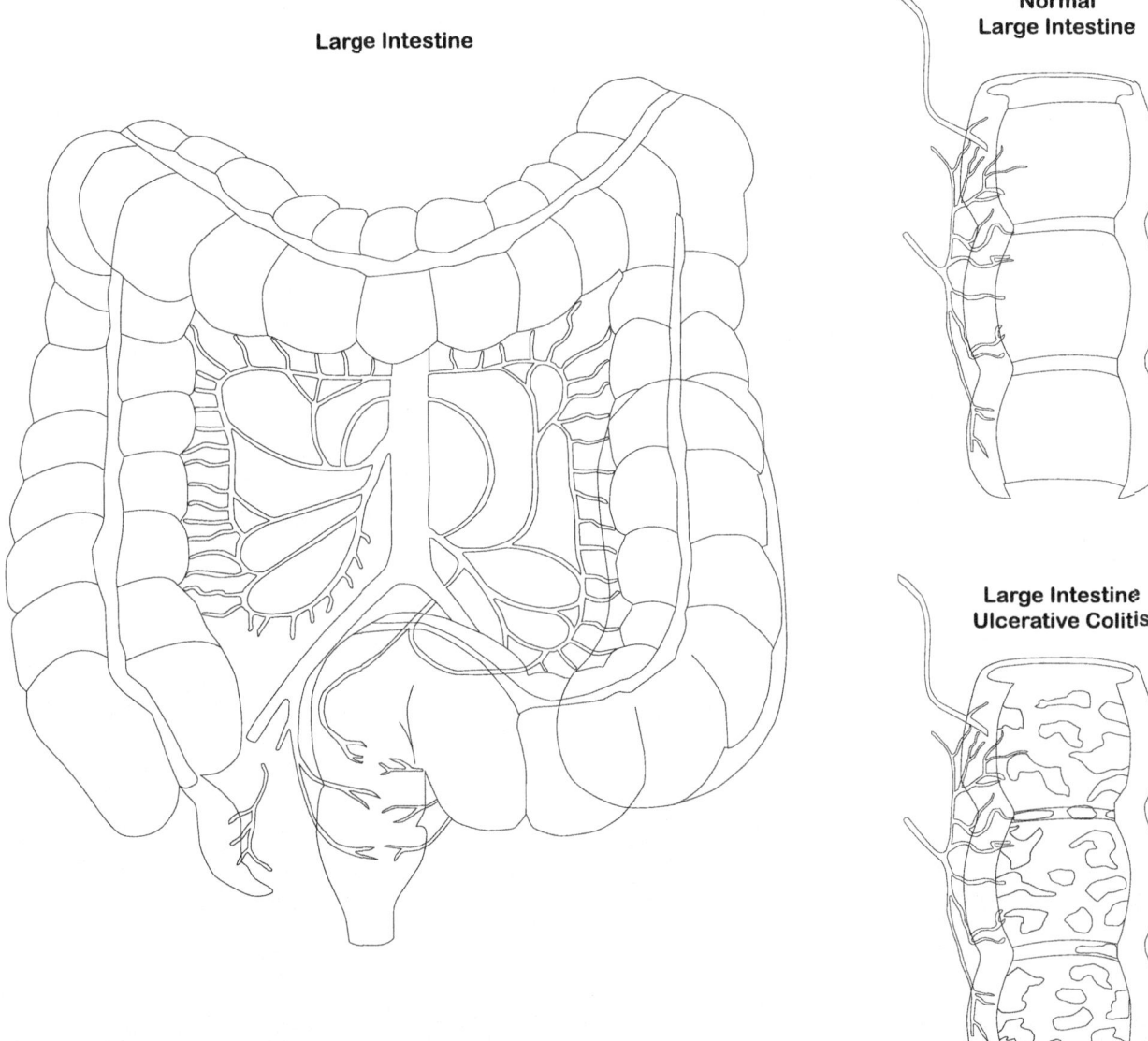

Irritable Bowel Syndrome
IBS

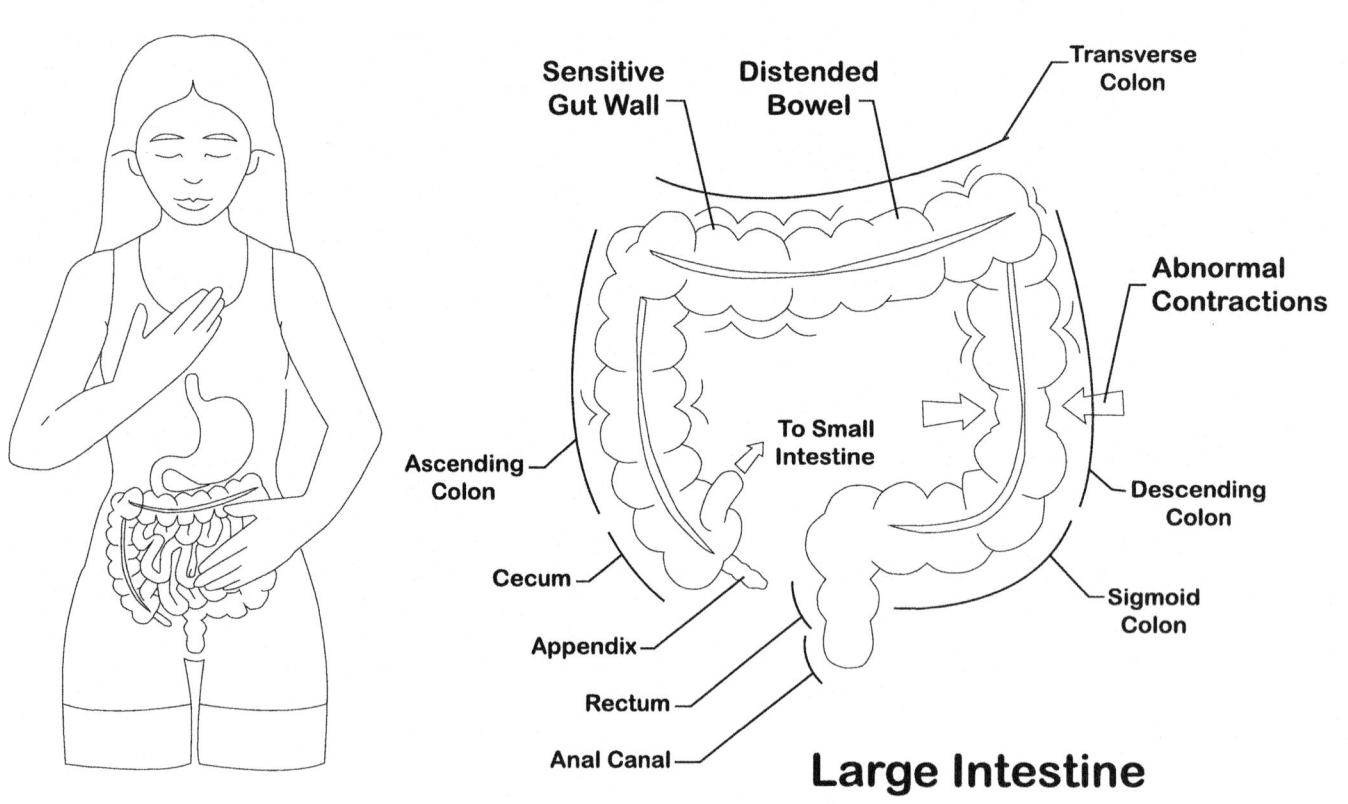

Diverticulitis

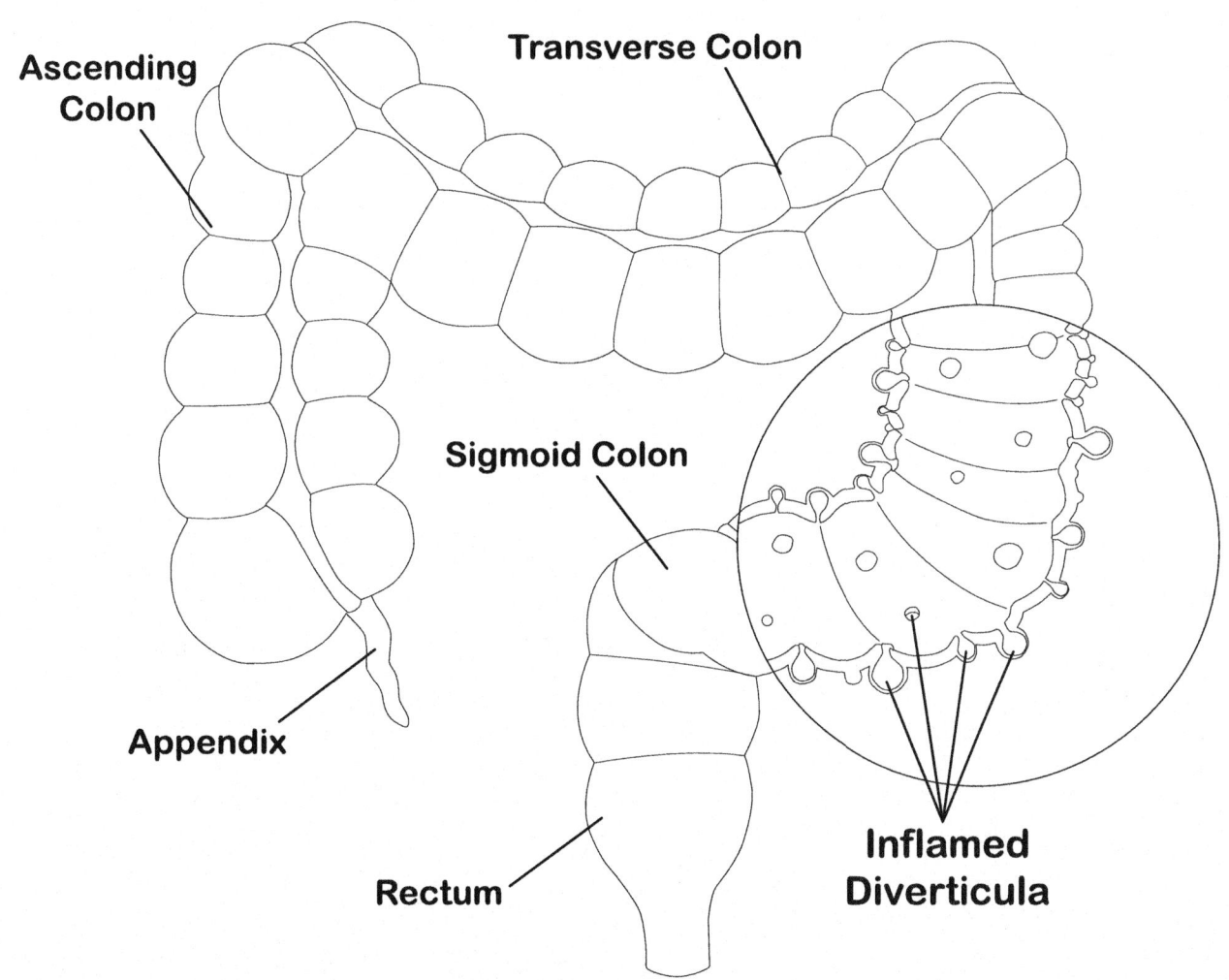

Cirrhosis

Healthy Liver

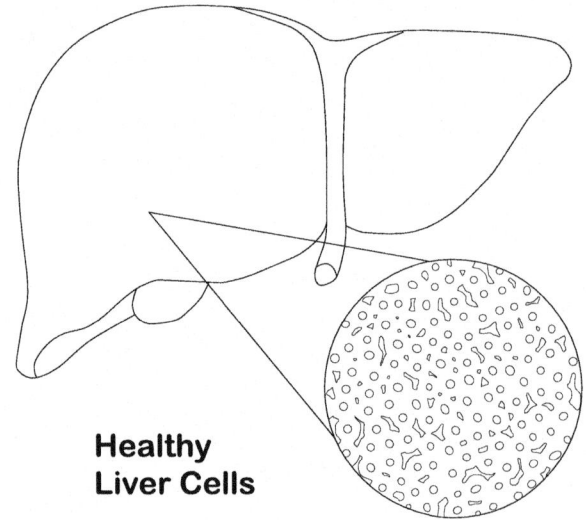

Healthy Liver Cells

Cirrhosis

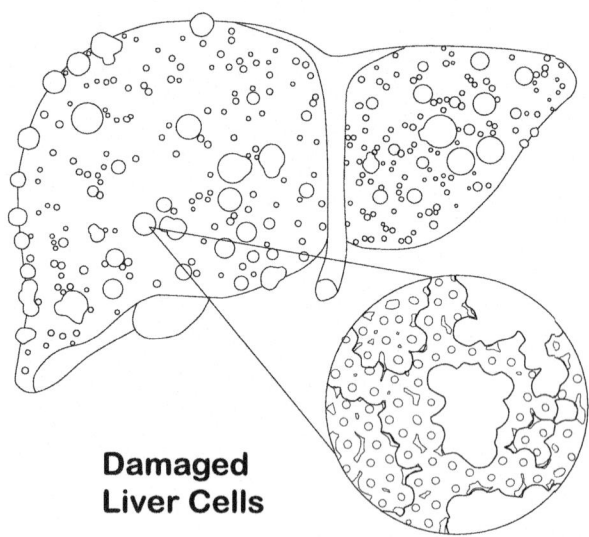

Damaged Liver Cells

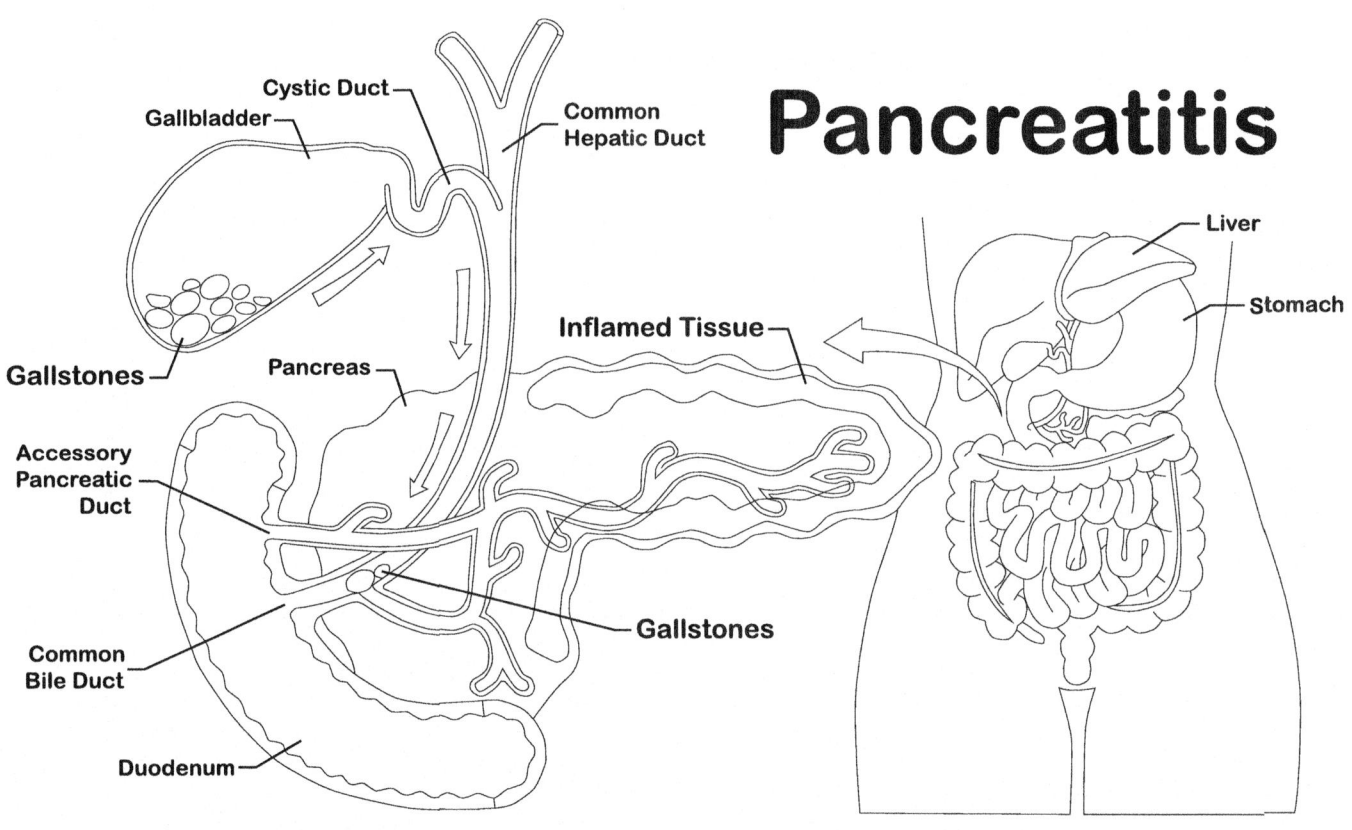

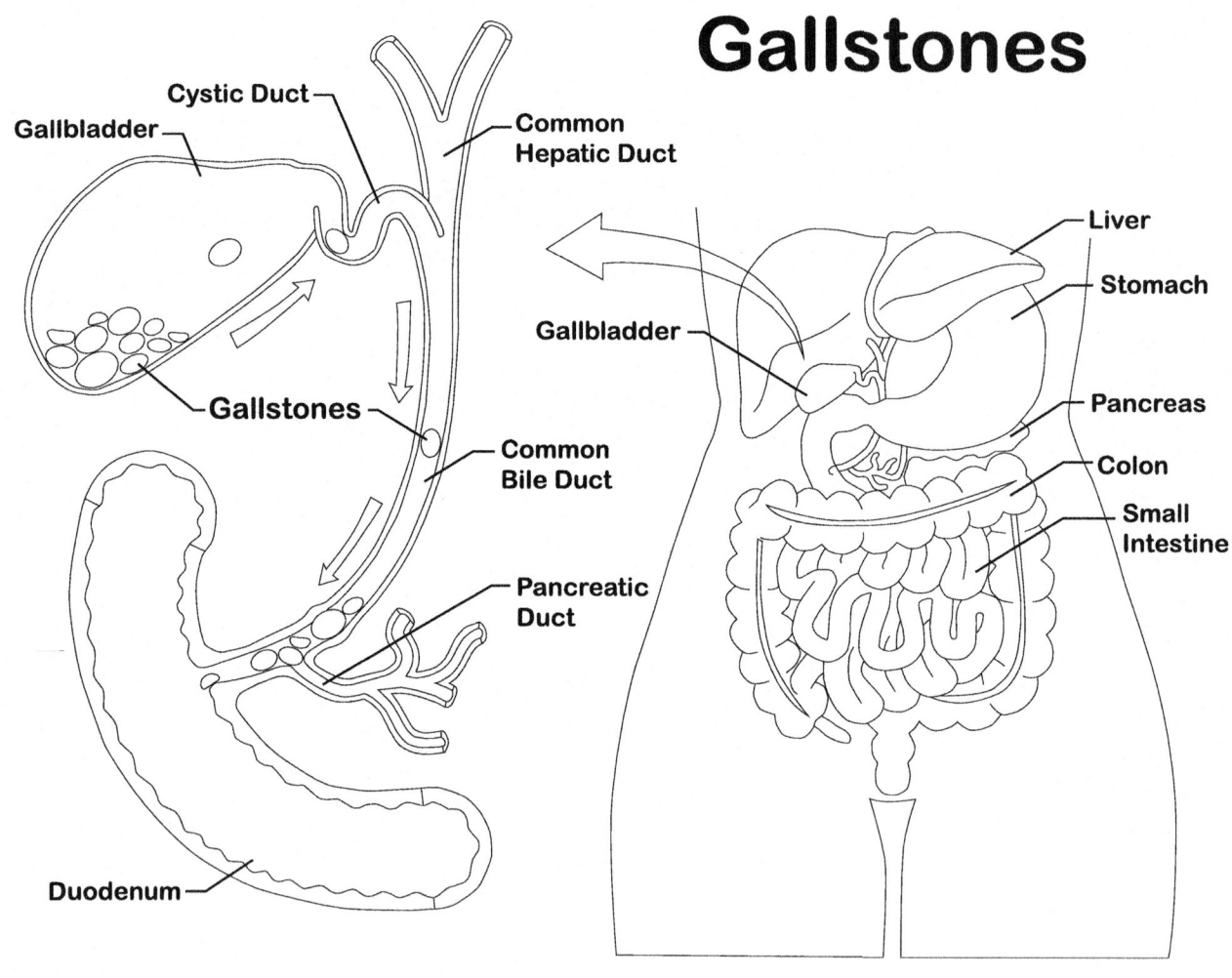

Colorectal Cancer

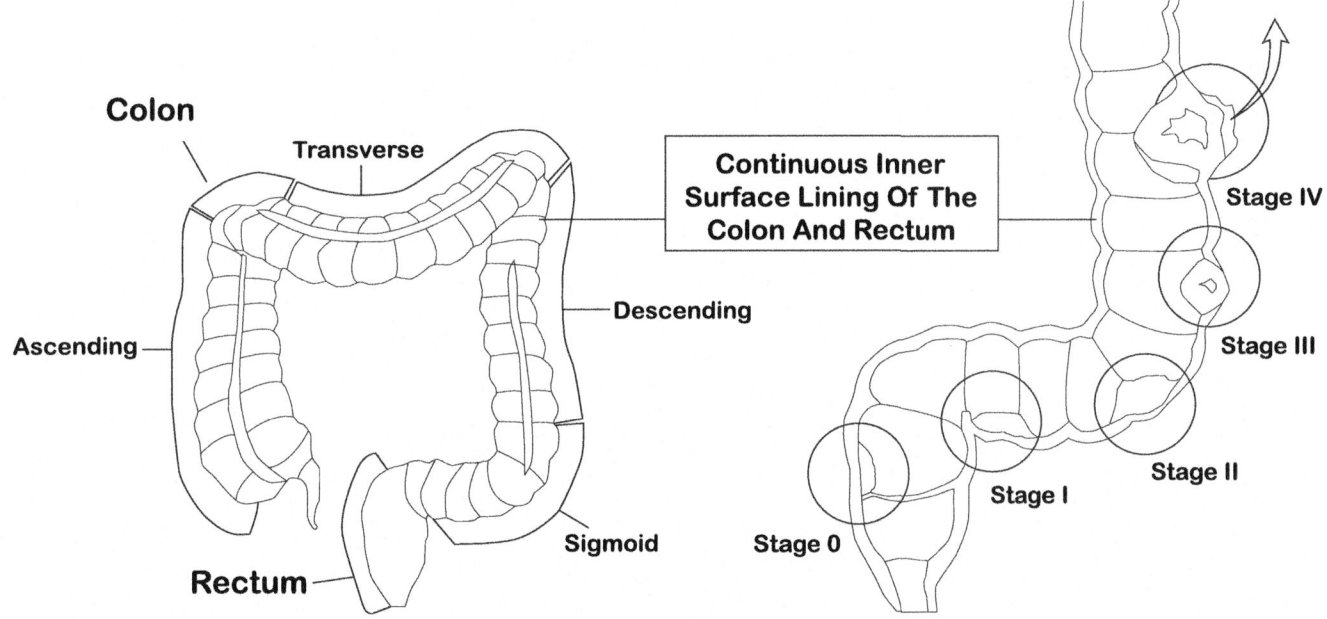

Meningitis

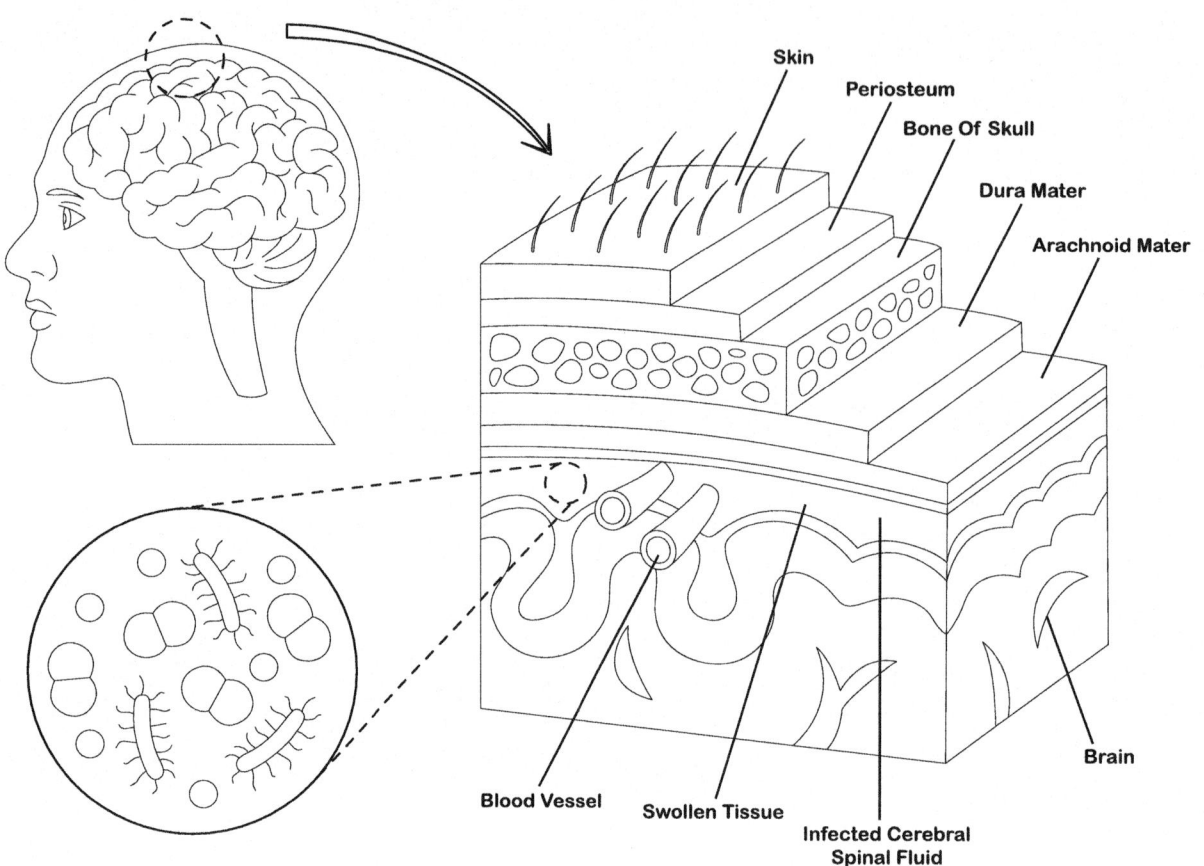

Viral Encephalitis

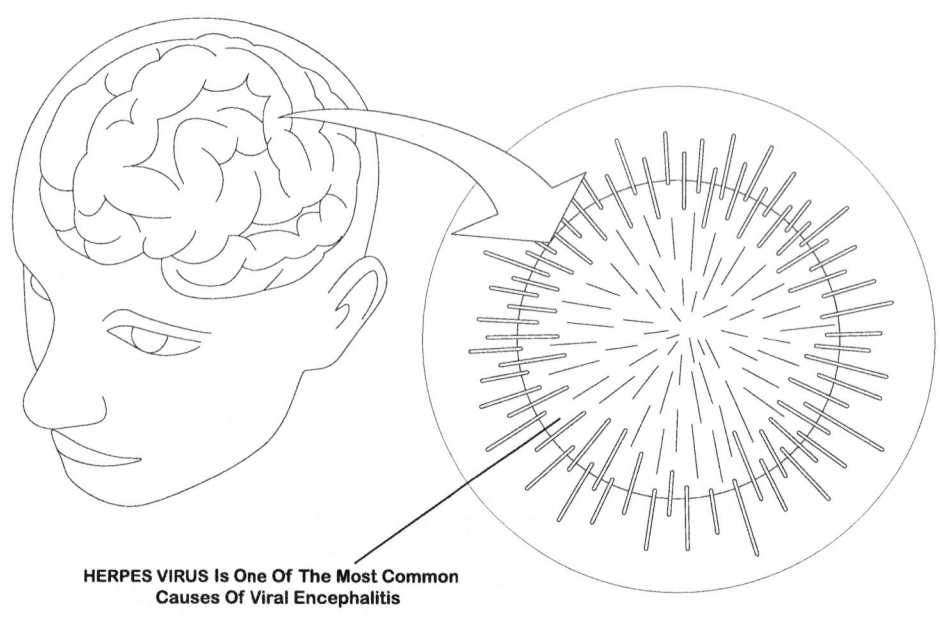

HERPES VIRUS Is One Of The Most Common Causes Of Viral Encephalitis

Brain Abscess

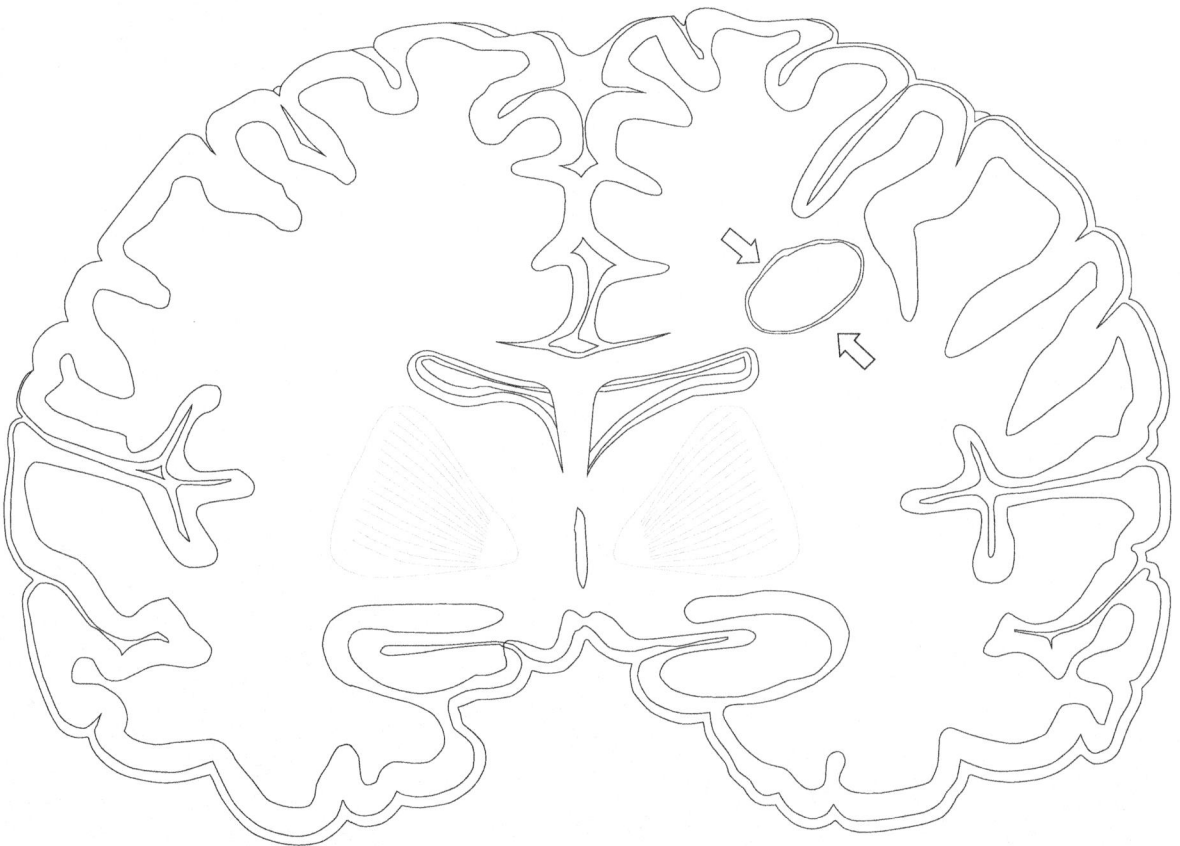

Inflammation and Collection Of Infected Material

Cerebral Malaria

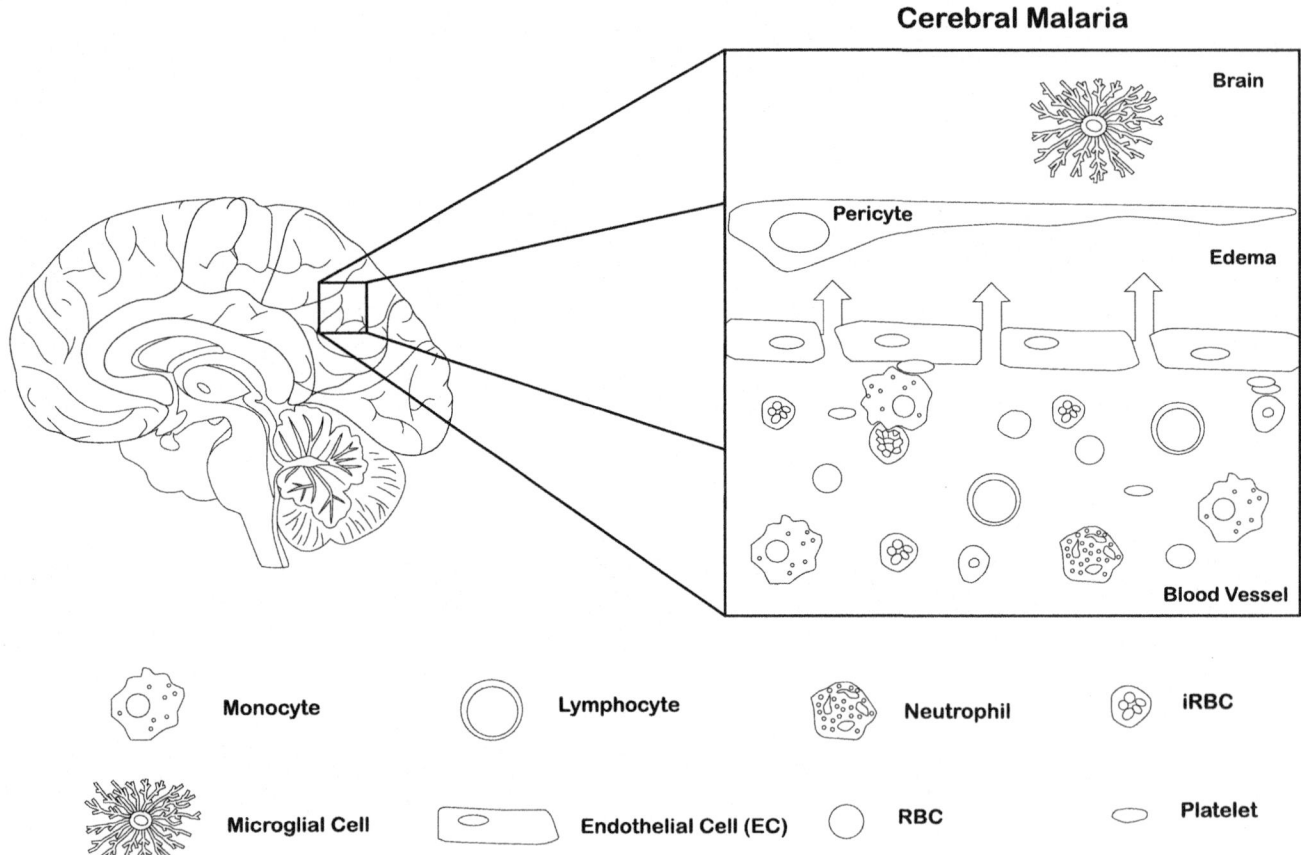

Types Of Brain Stroke

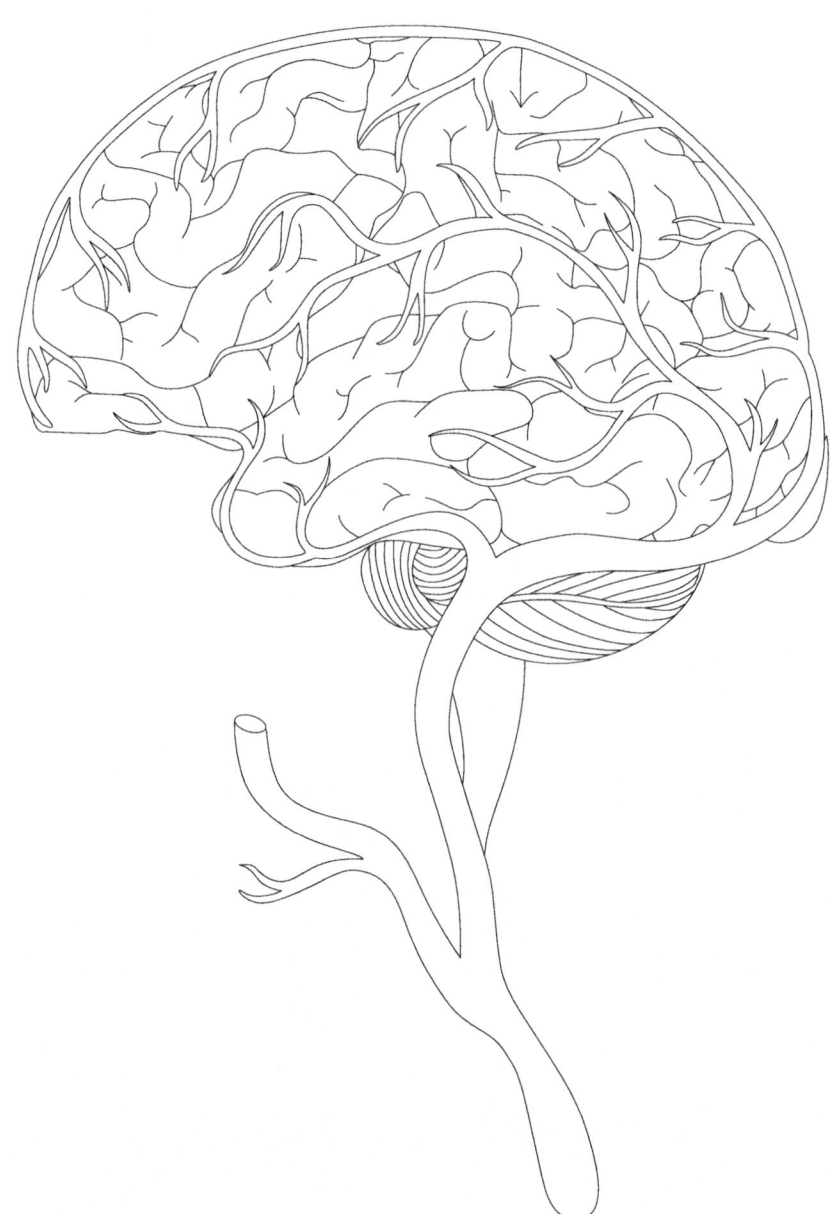

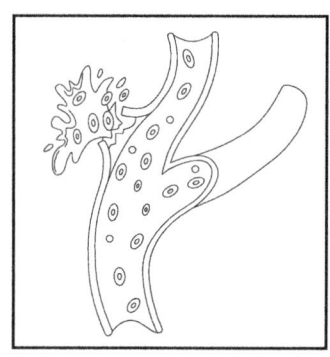
Hemorrhagic

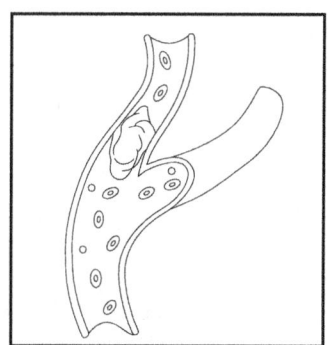
Ischemic

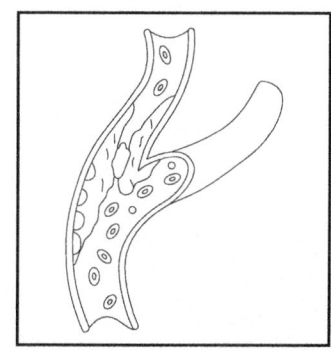
Atherosclerosis

Alzheimer's Disease

Healthy Brain
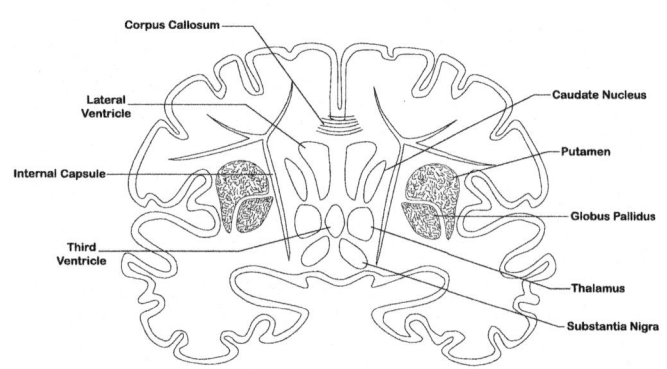

Alzheimer's
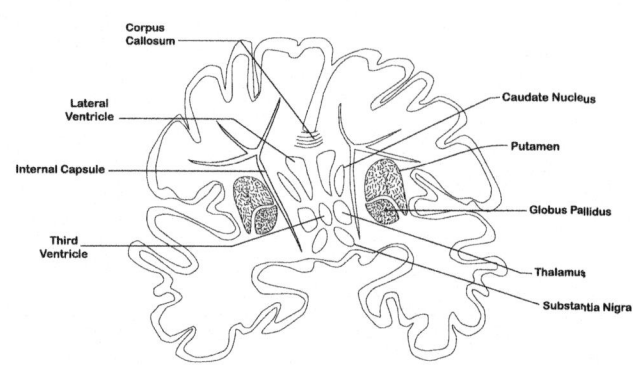

Parkinson's Disease

Healthy Brain
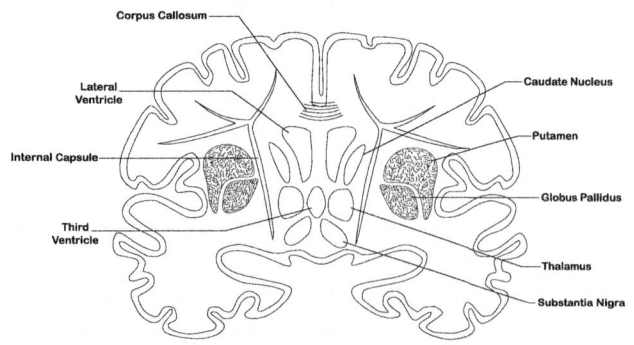

Parkinson's Disease Brain
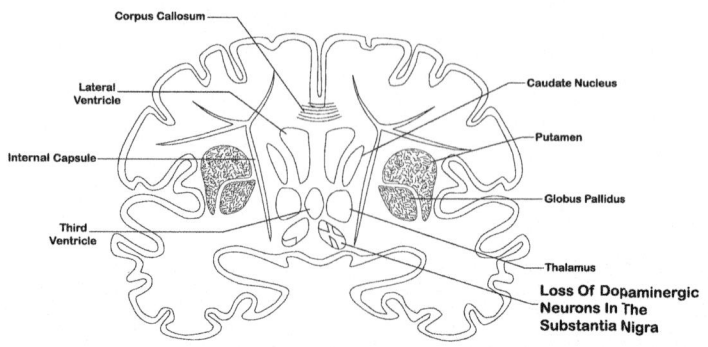

Huntington's Disease

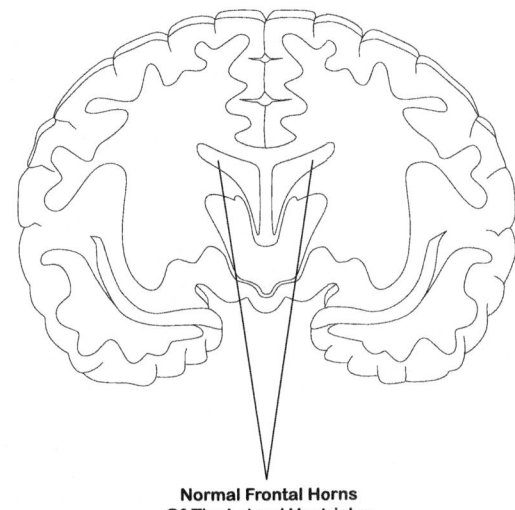
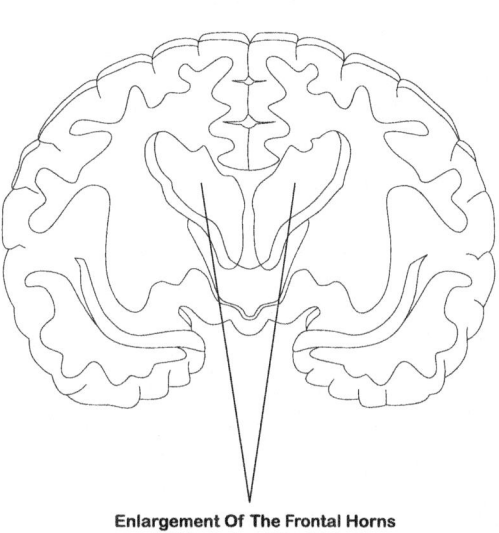

Multiple Sclerosis

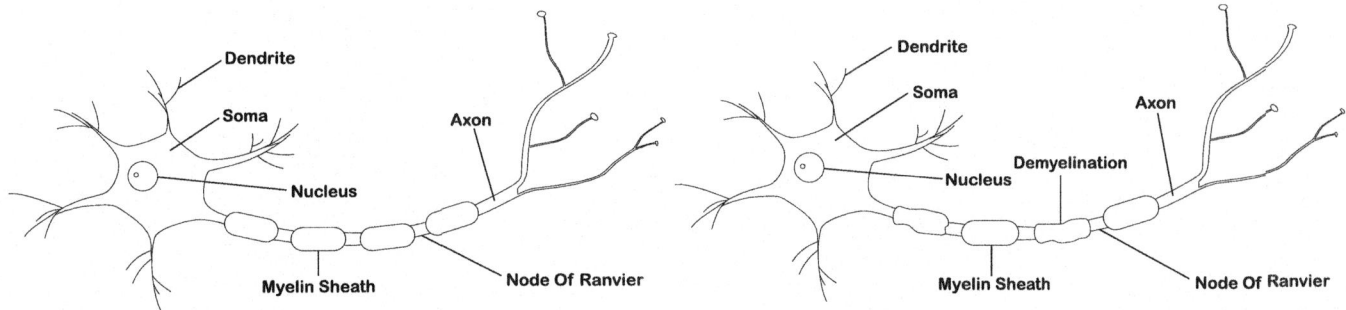

Epilepsy

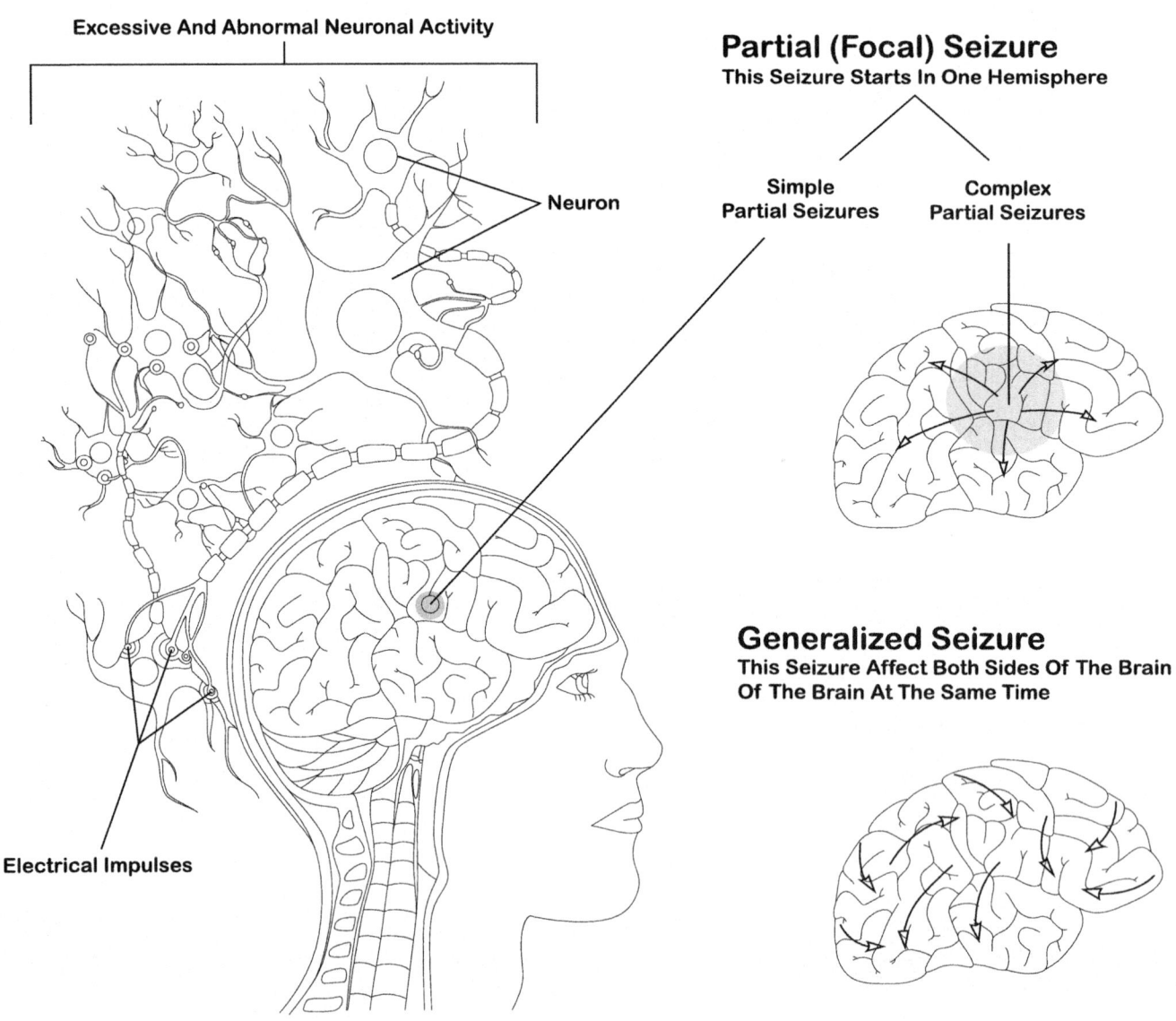

Amyotrophic Lateral Sclerosis (ALS)

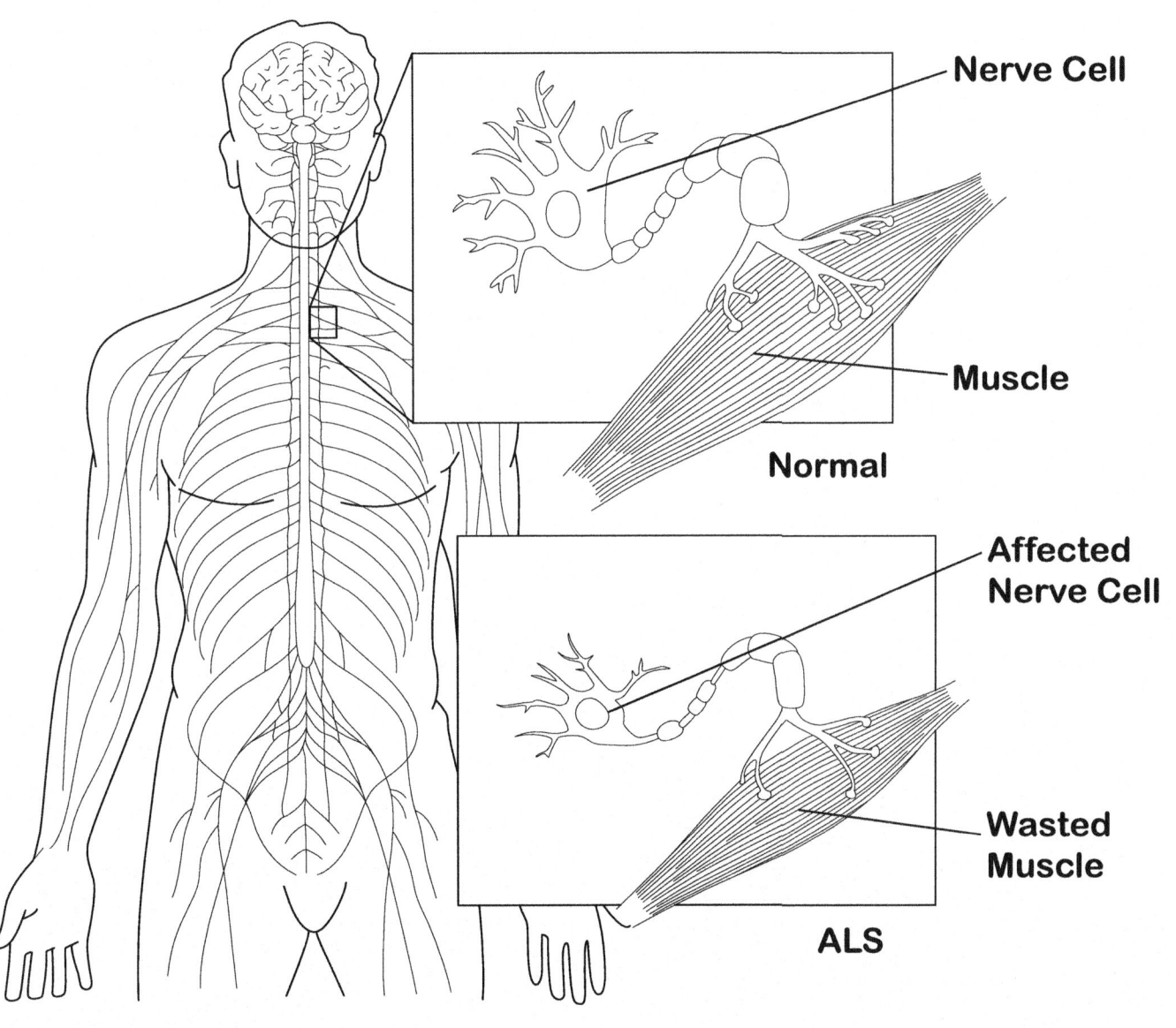

Neuropathy
Nerve Damage

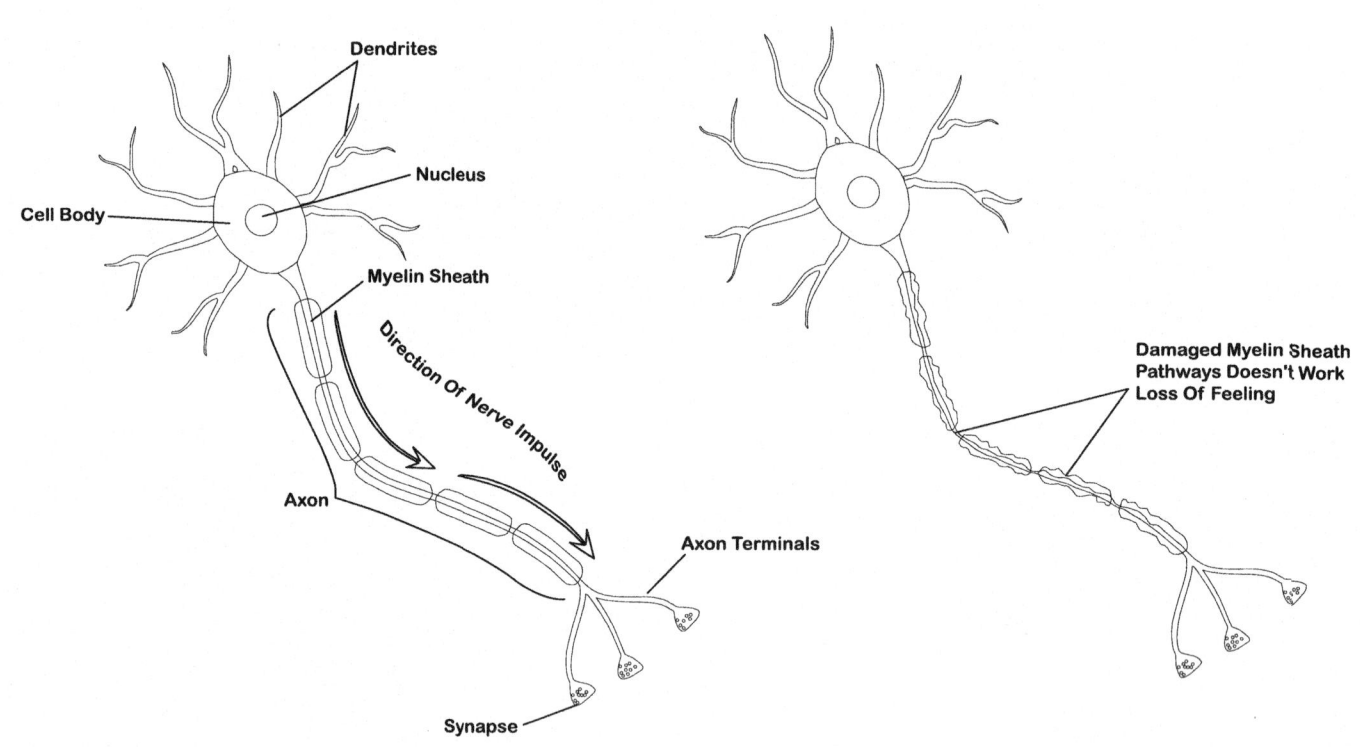

Healthy Nerve Cell   Unhealthy Nerve Cell

Urinary Tract Infection - UTI

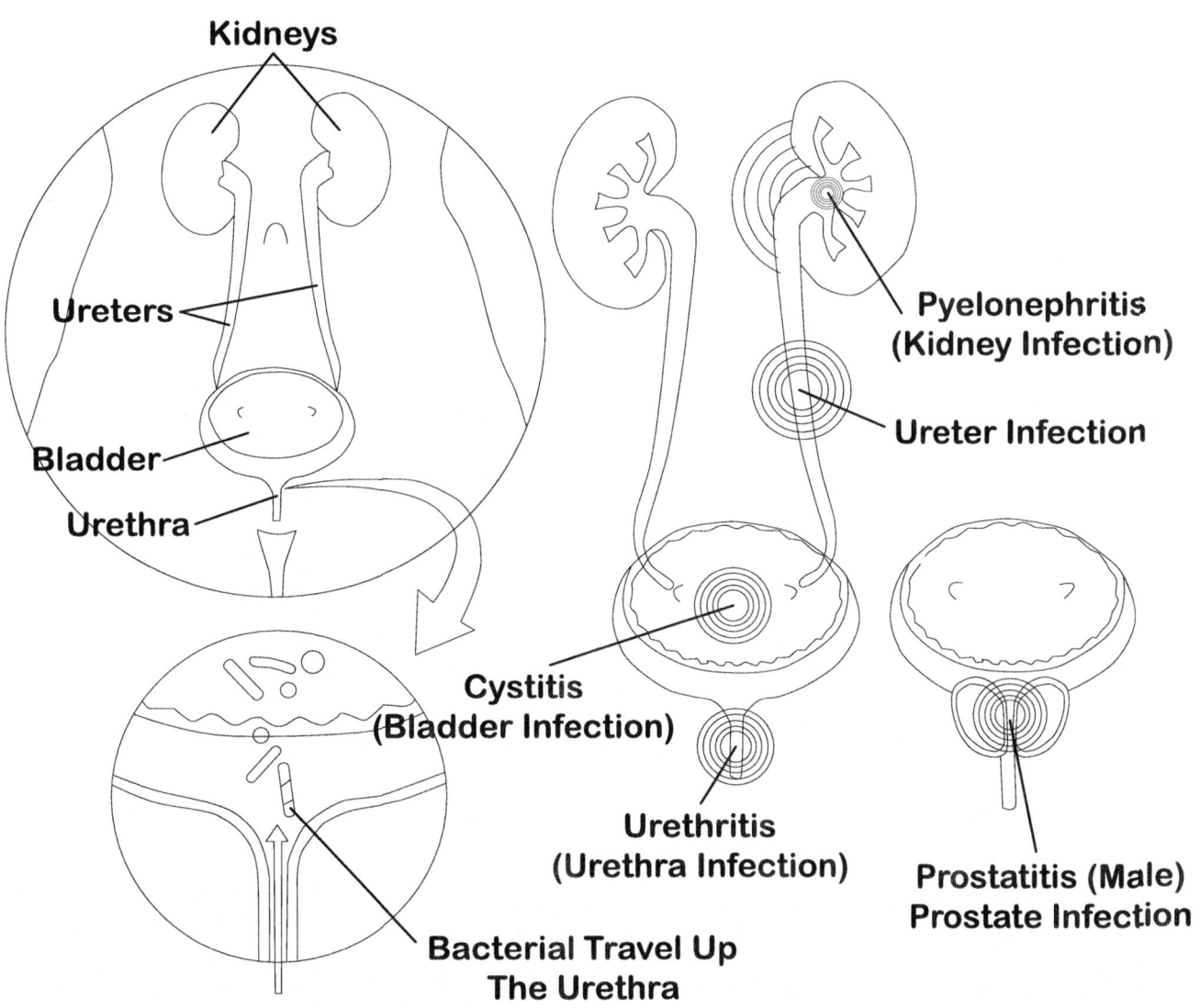

Kidney Stones

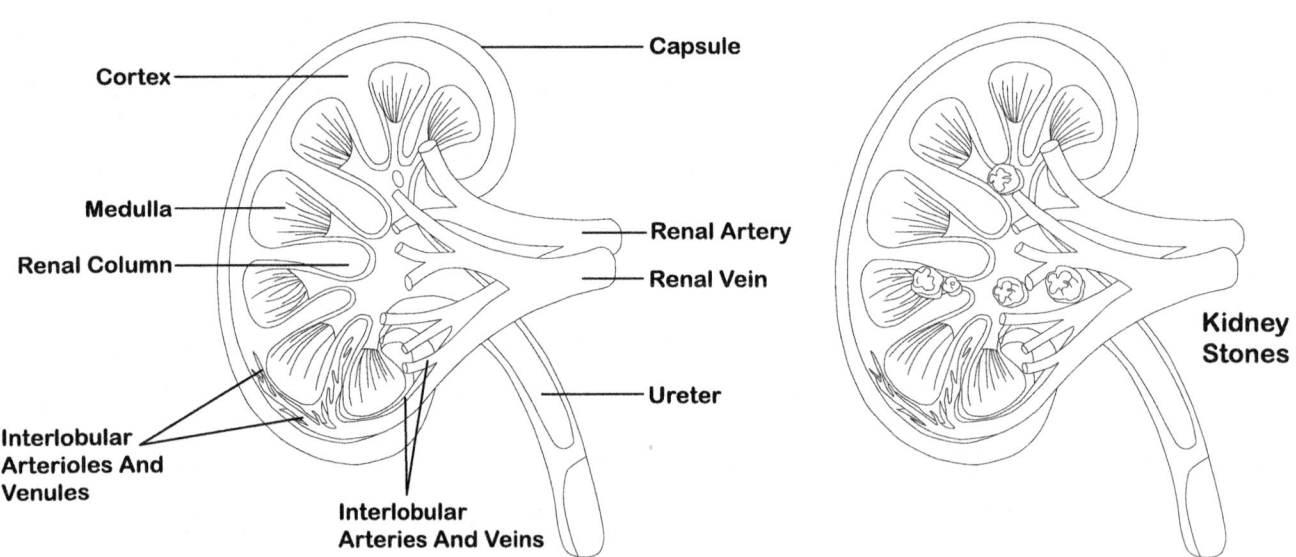

Types Of Incontinence
(Incontinentia Vesicae)

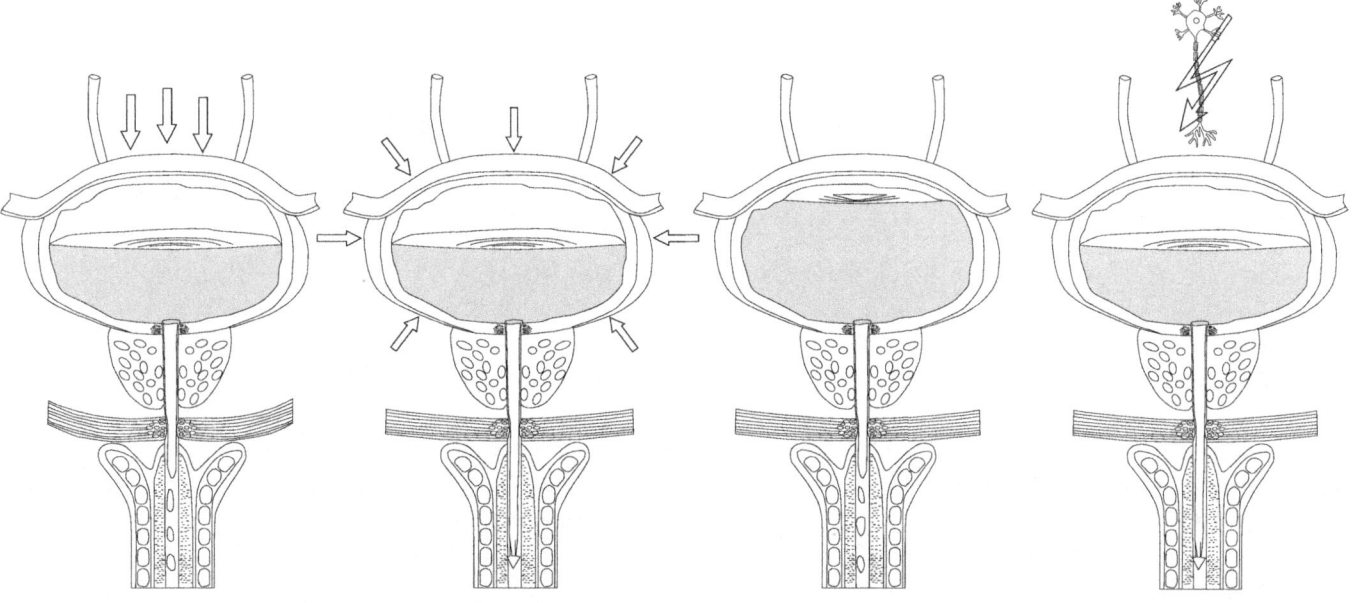

Stress Incontinence
Due To Increased Abdominal Pressure Under Stress (Weak Pelvic Floor Muscles)

Urge Incontinence
Due To Involuntary Contraction Of The Bladder Muscles

Overflow Incontinence
Due To Blockage Of The Urethra

Neurogenic Incontinence
Due To Disturbed Function Of The Nervous System

Benign Prostatic Hyperplasia

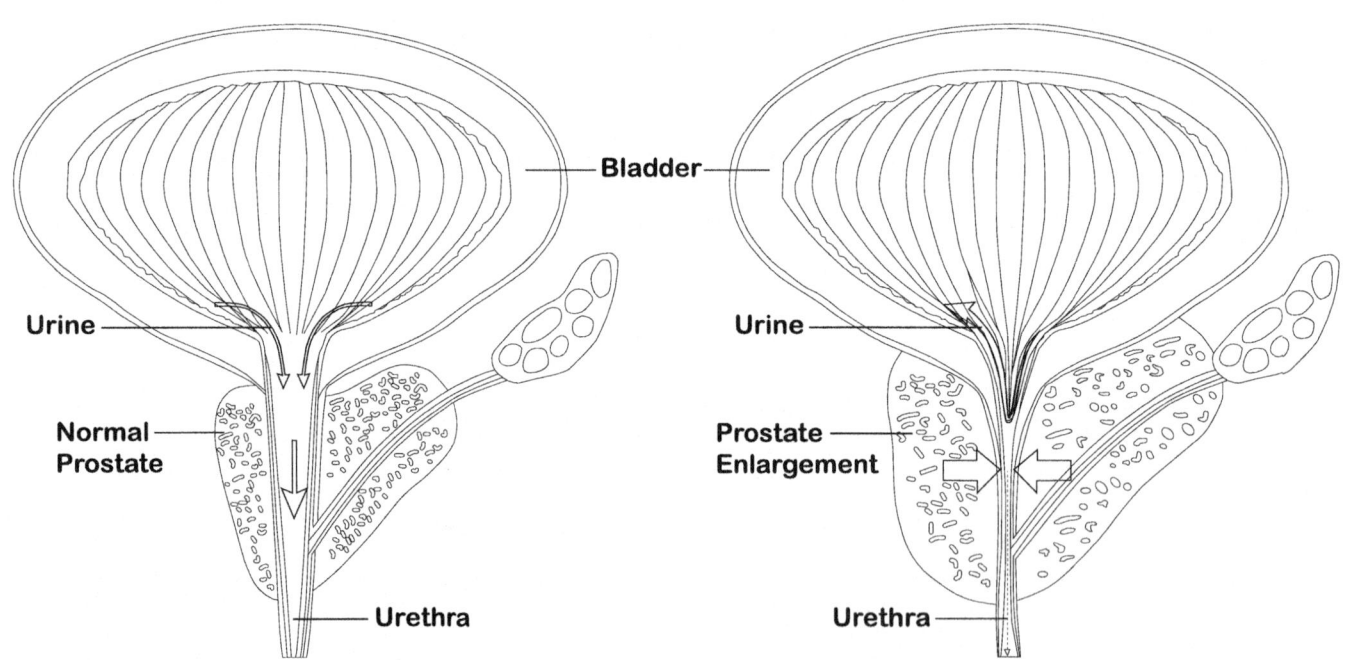

Prostatitis

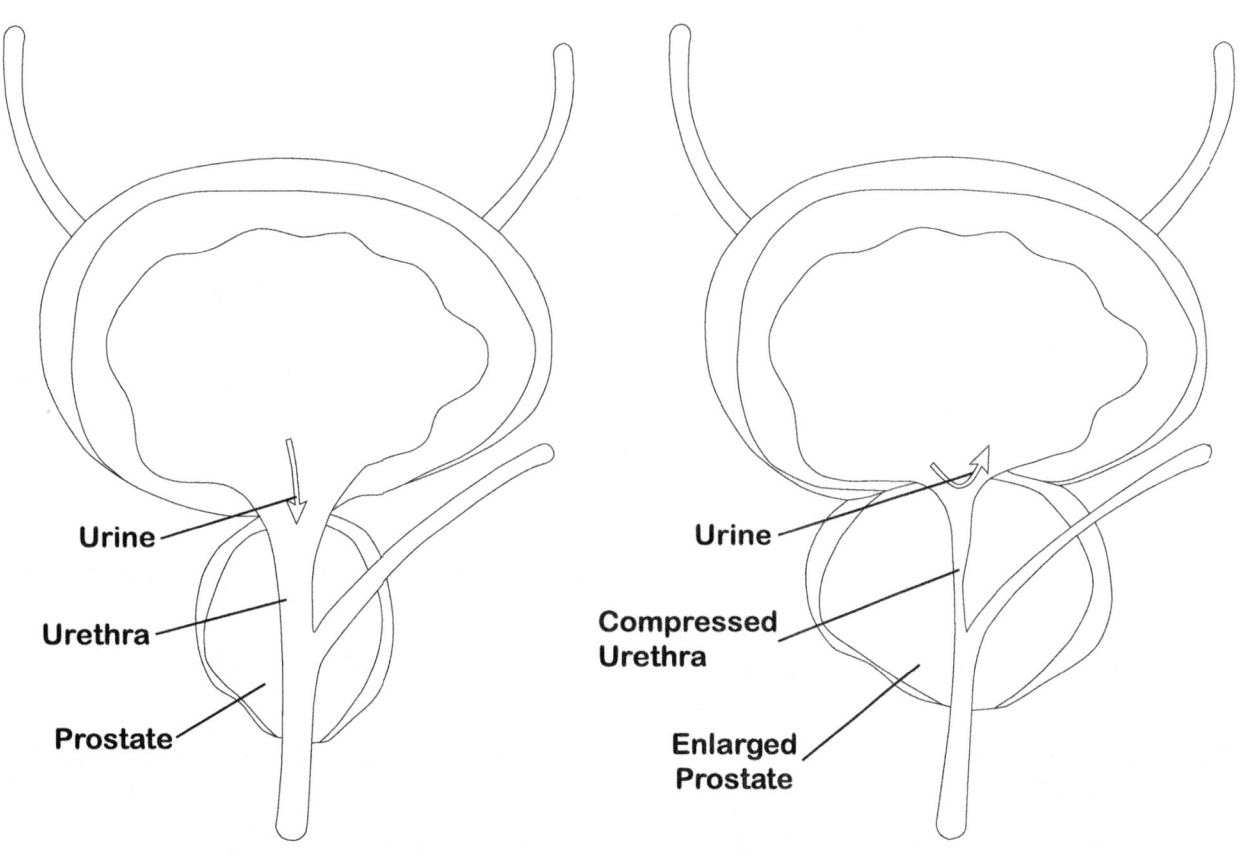

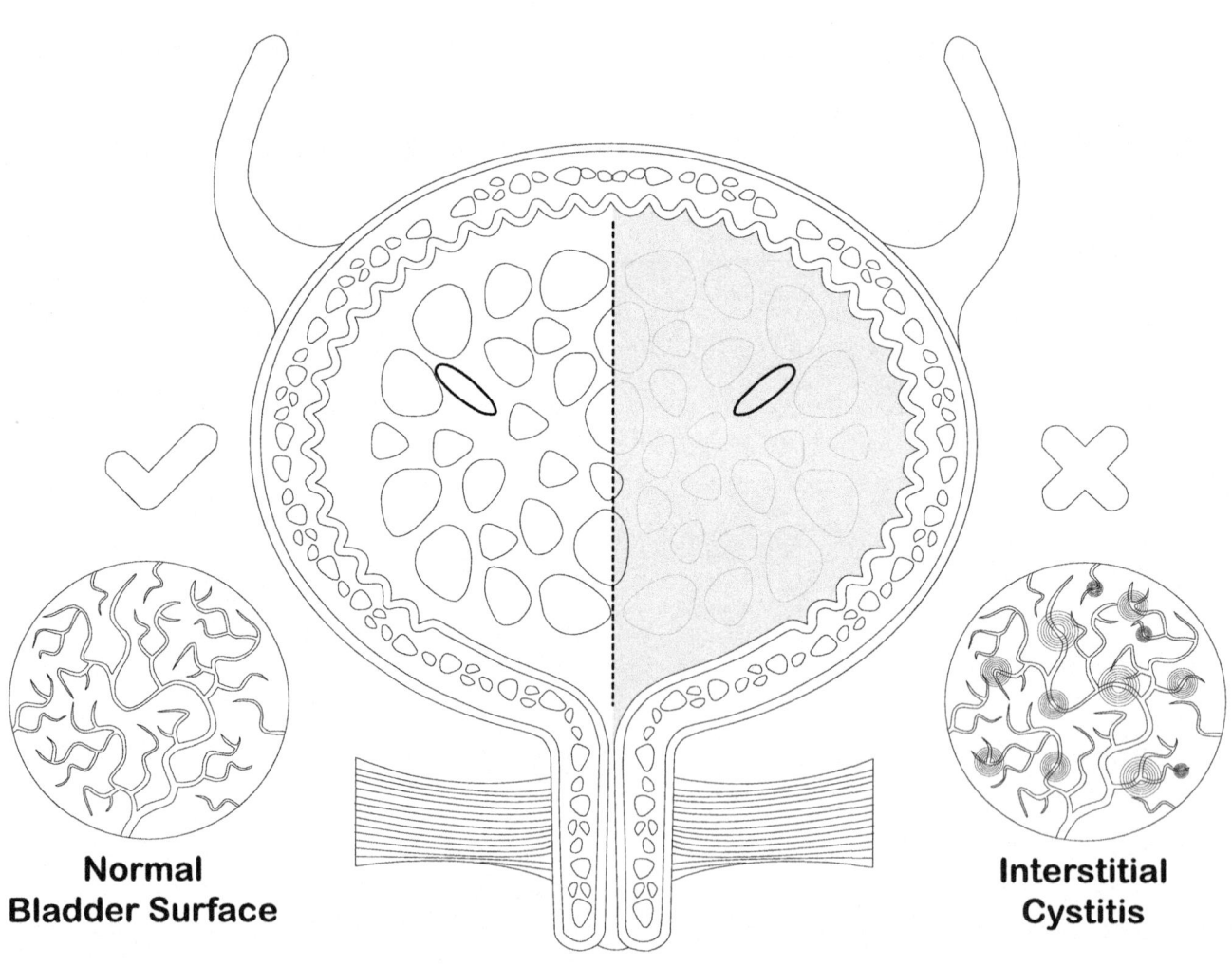

Erectile Dysfunction

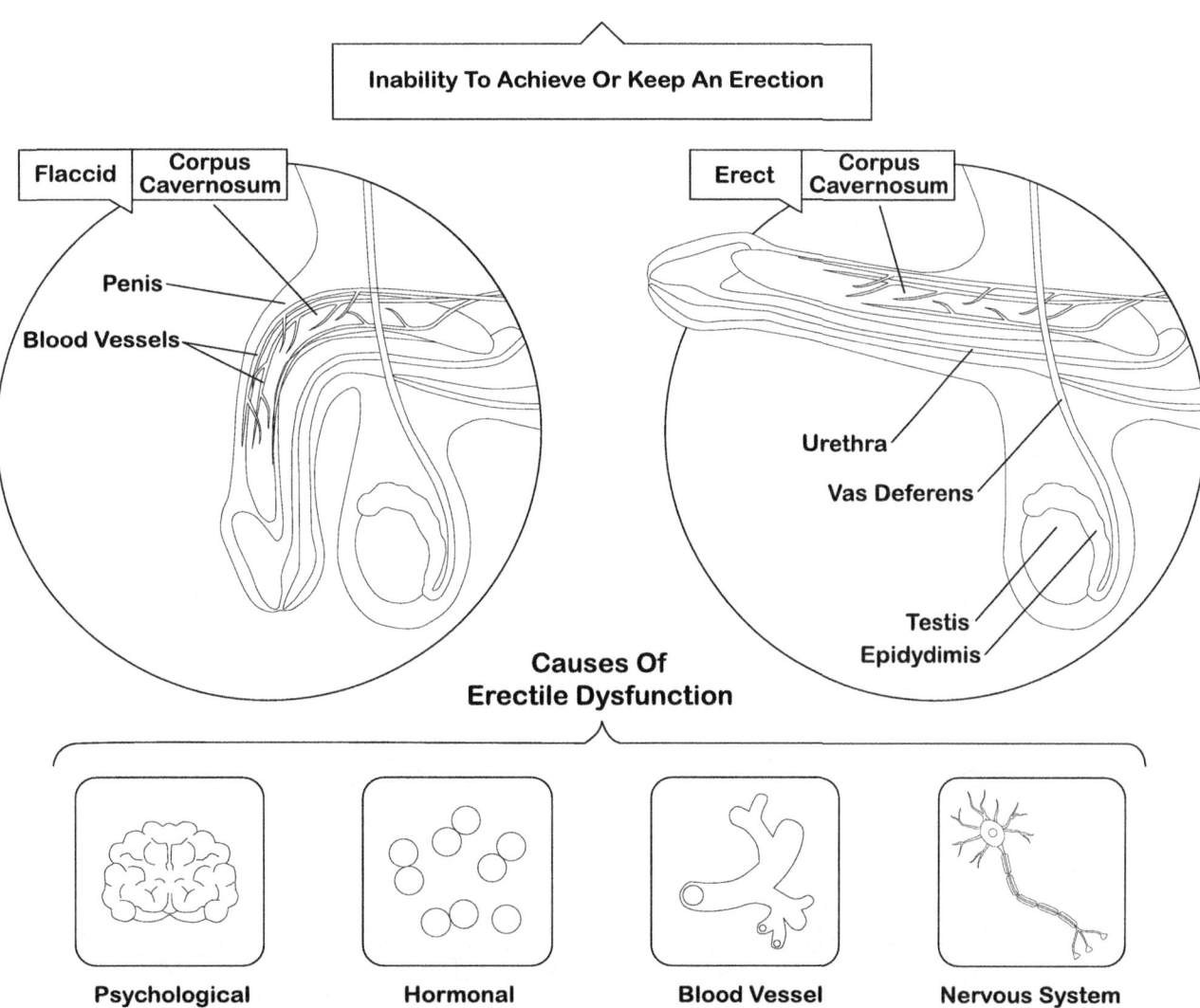

Polycystic Kidney

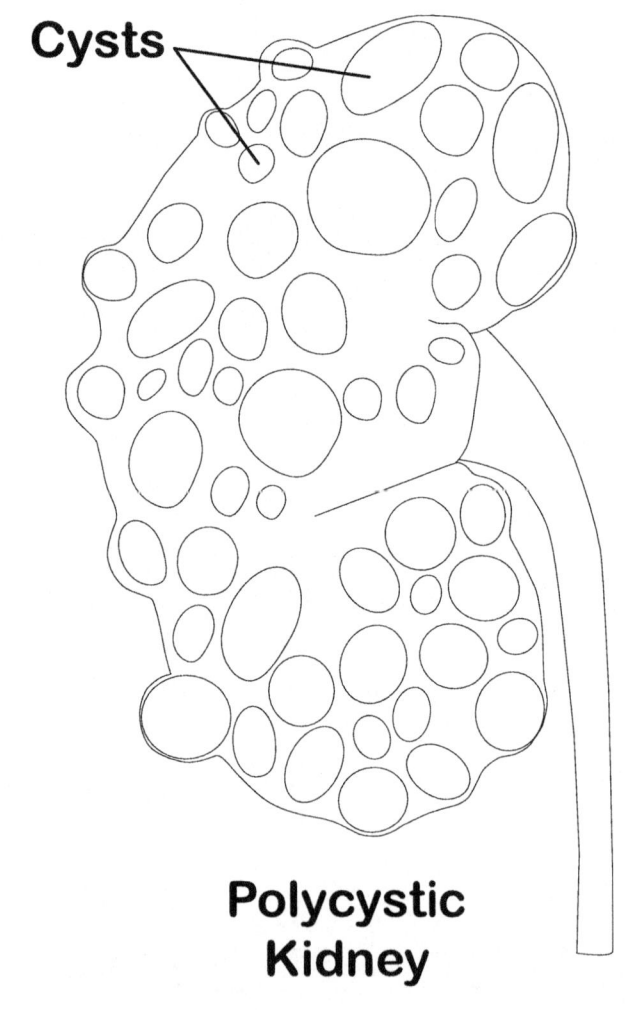

Polycystic Kidney

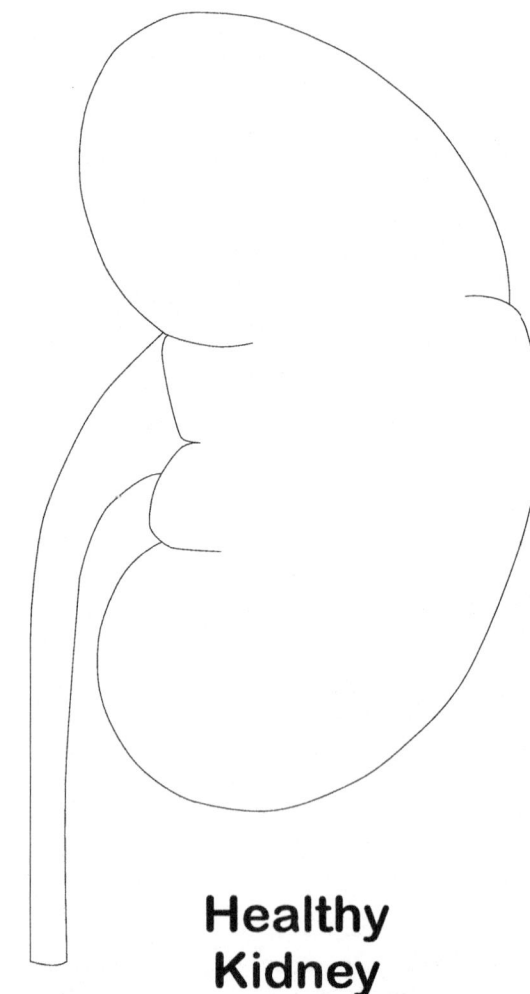

Healthy Kidney

Endometriosis

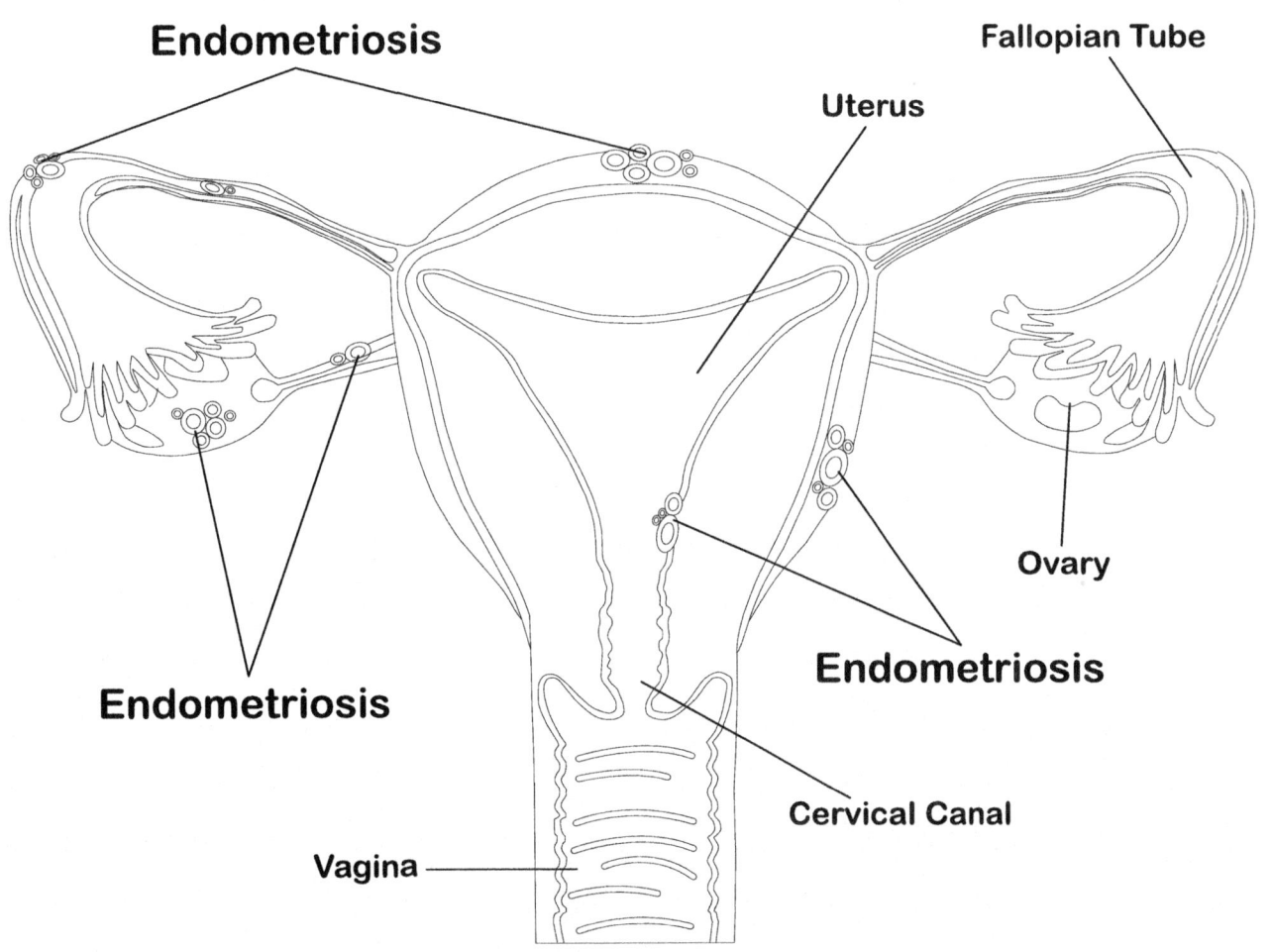

Pyelonephritis

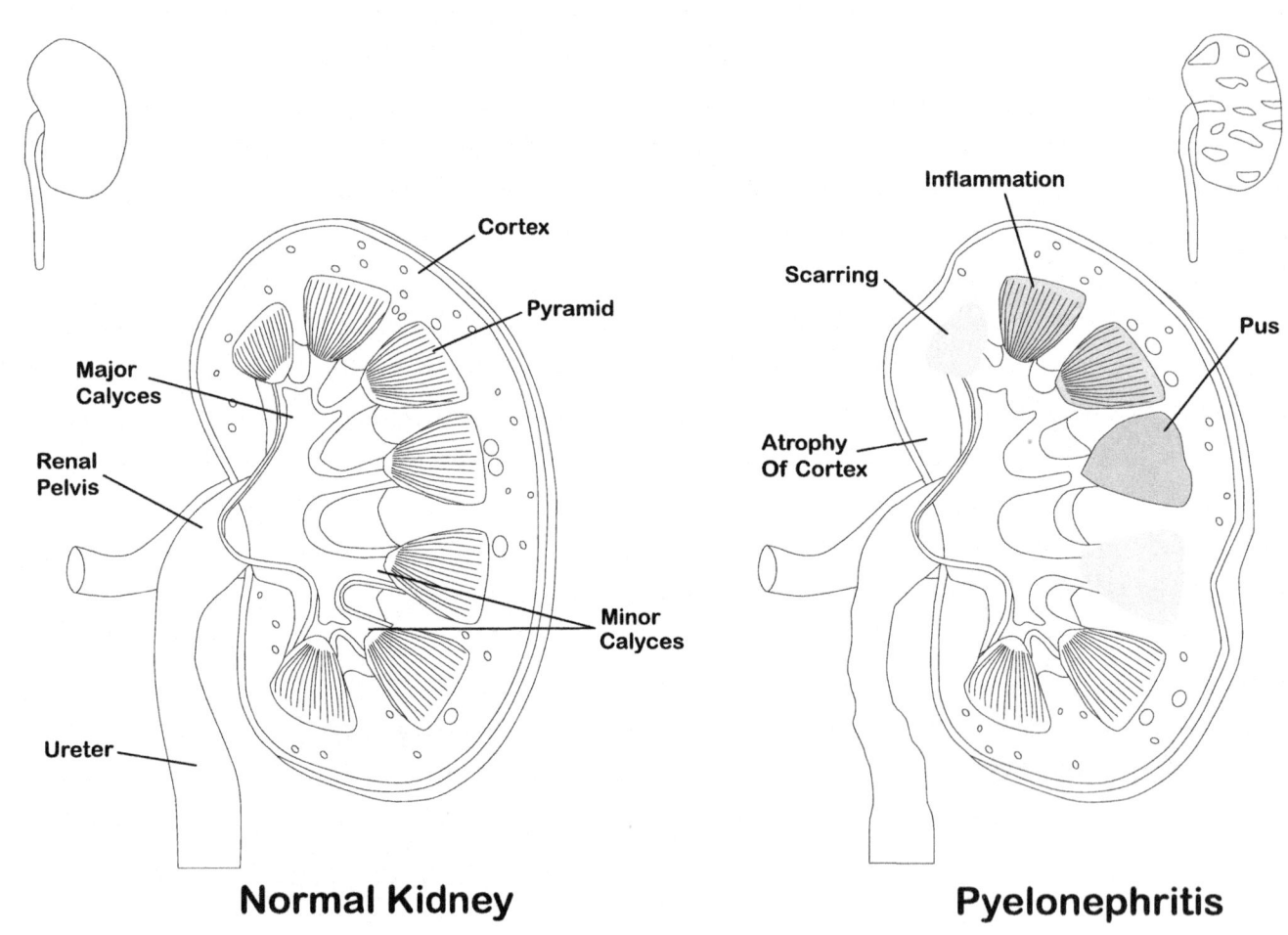

Genital Herpes

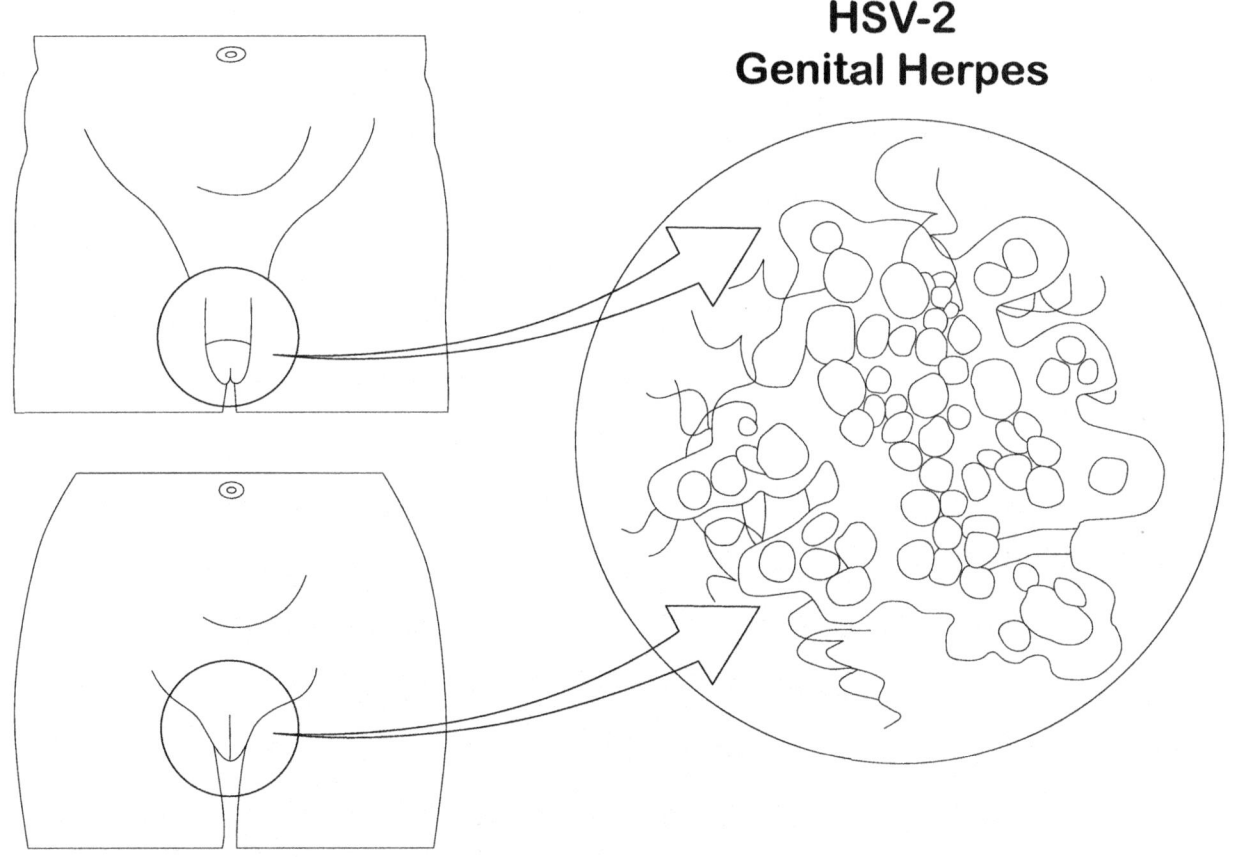

Vaginal Thrush
Vaginal Yeast Infection

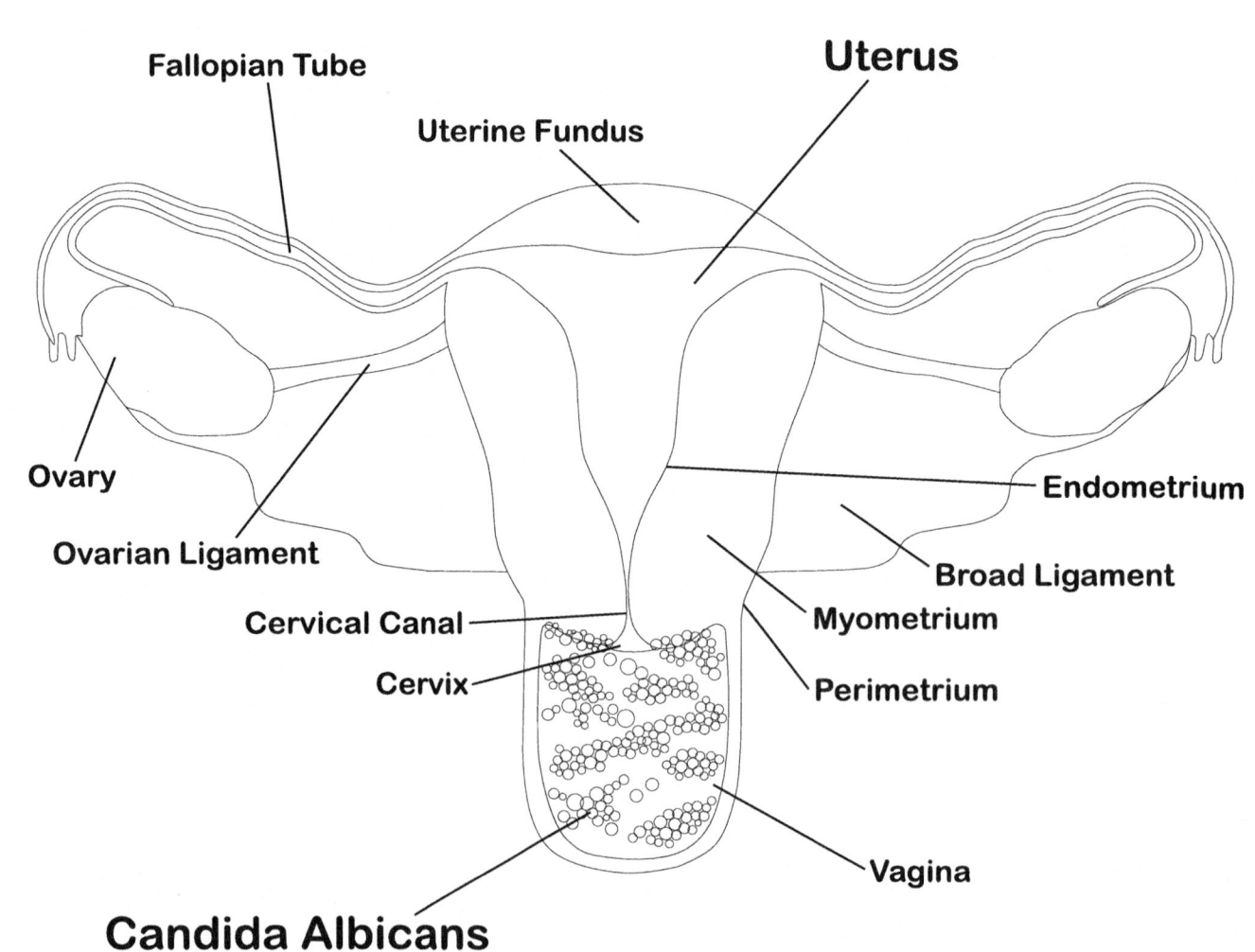

Pelvic Inflammatory Diseases

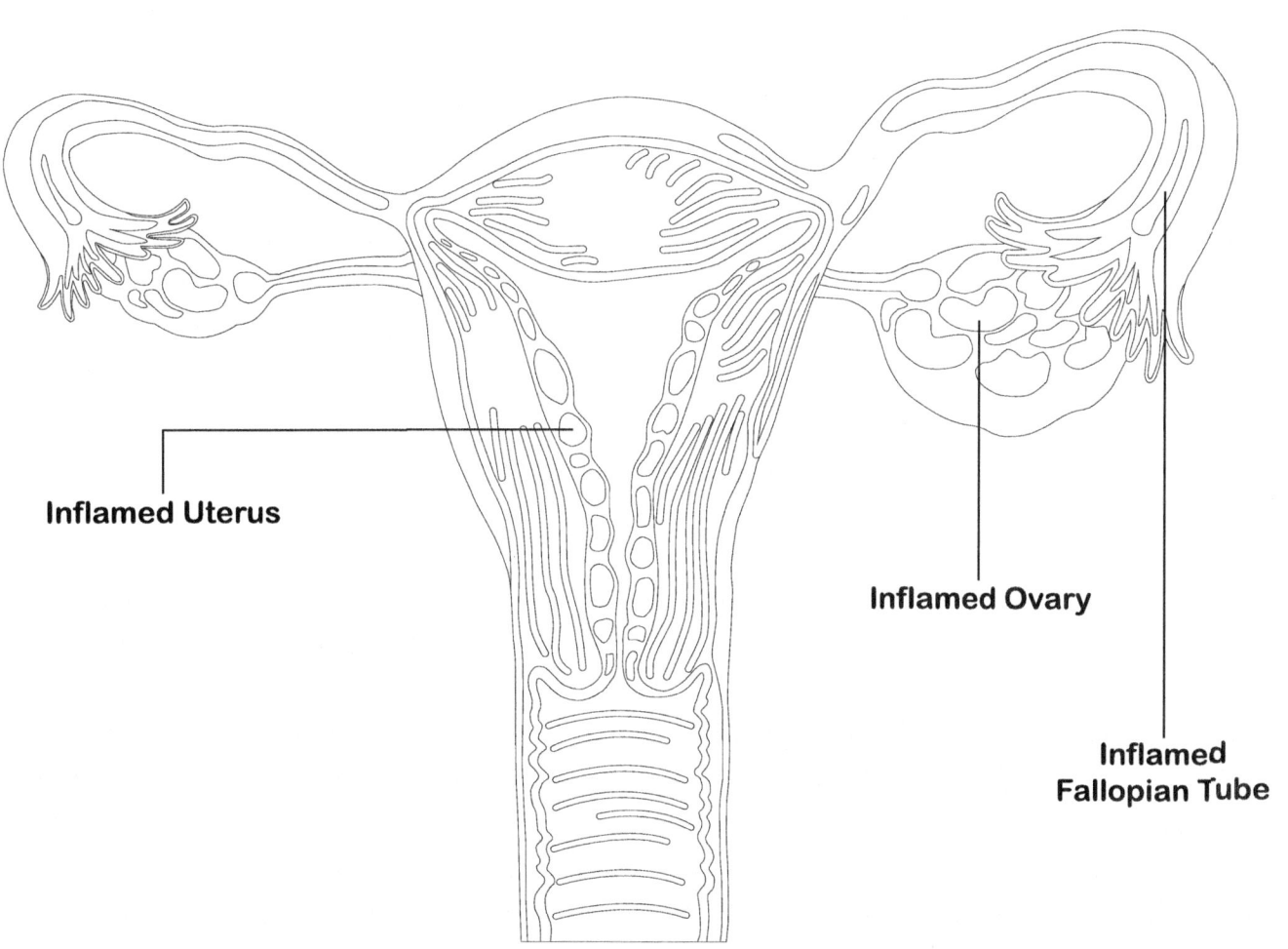

Inflamed Uterus

Inflamed Ovary

Inflamed Fallopian Tube

Impetigo

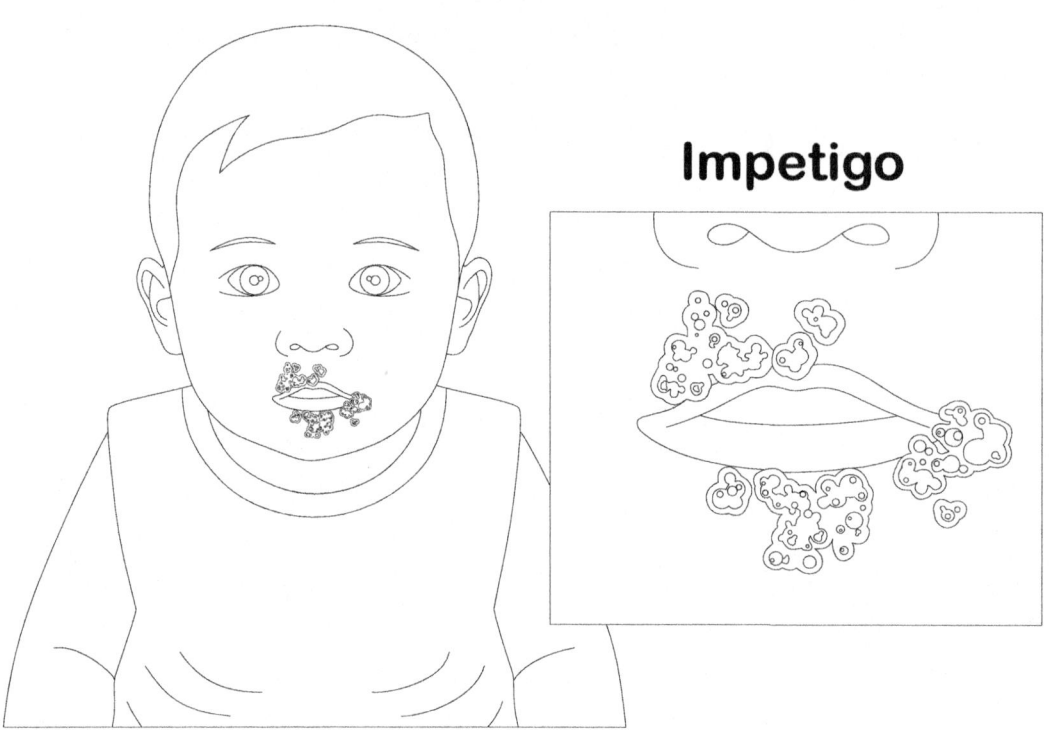

Cellulite

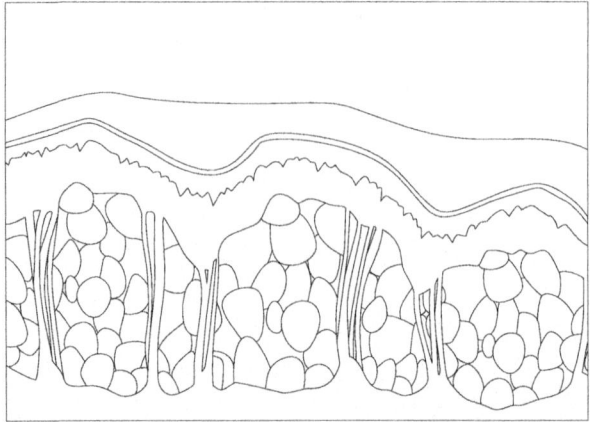
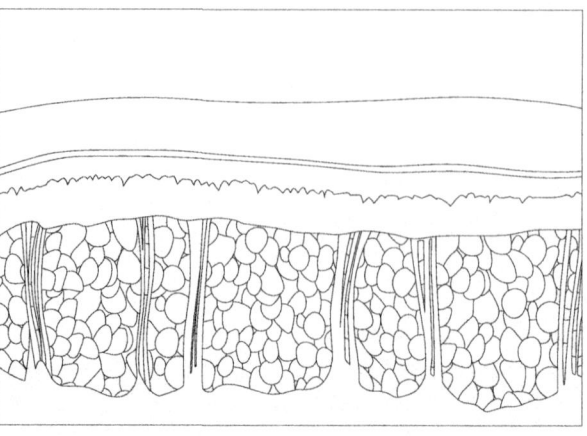

Athlete's Foot

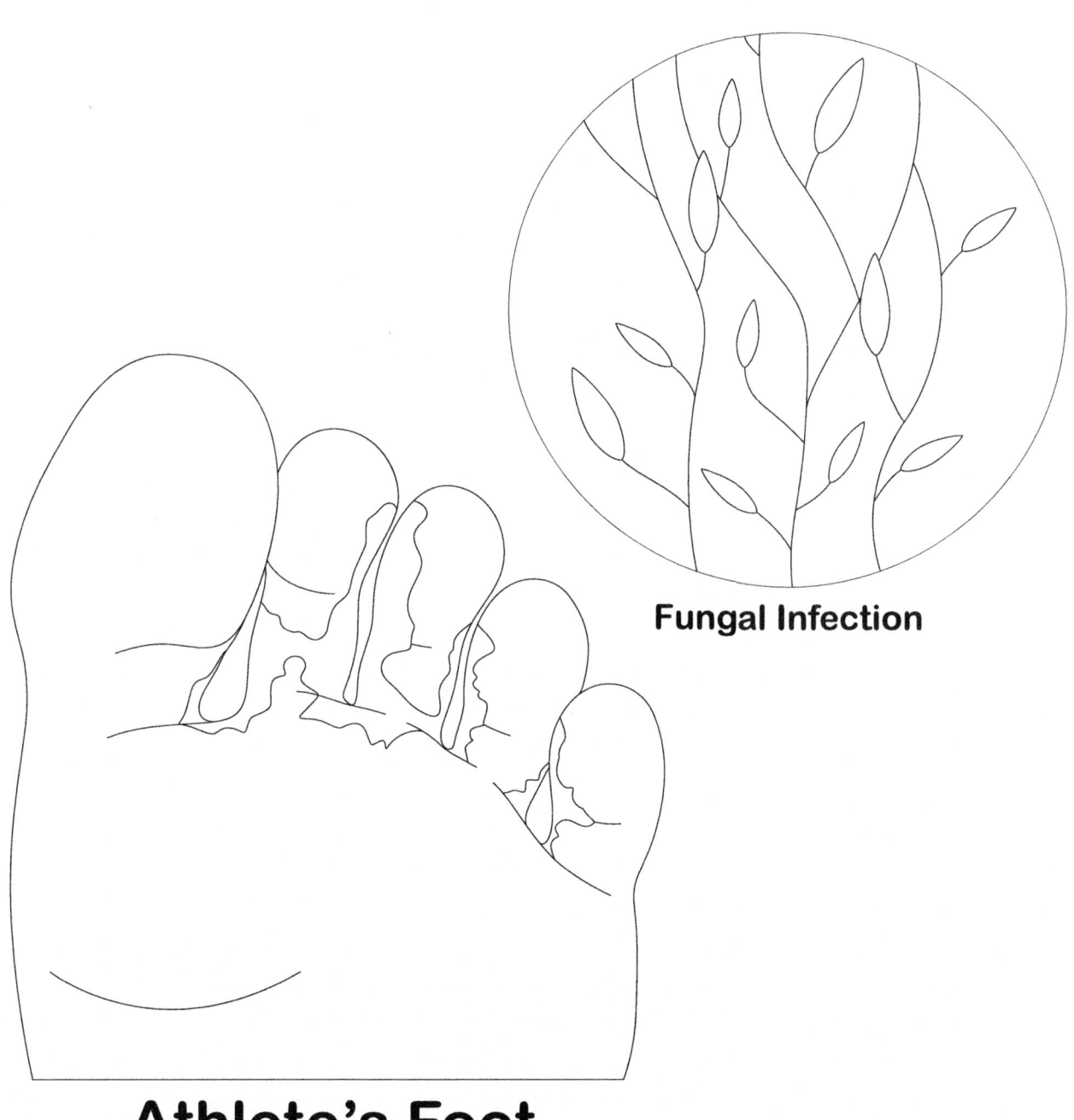

Fungal Infection

Athlete's Foot

Ringworm

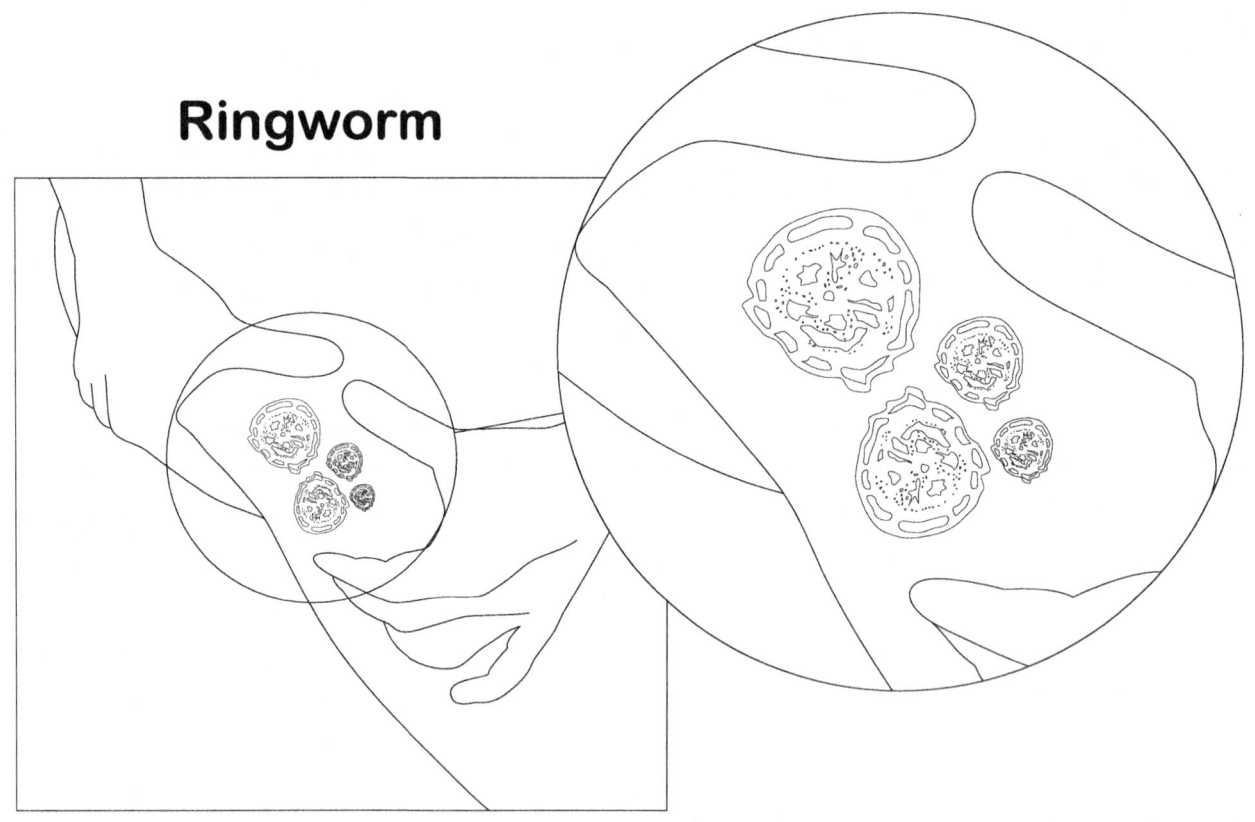

Three Kinds Of Fungal Infections

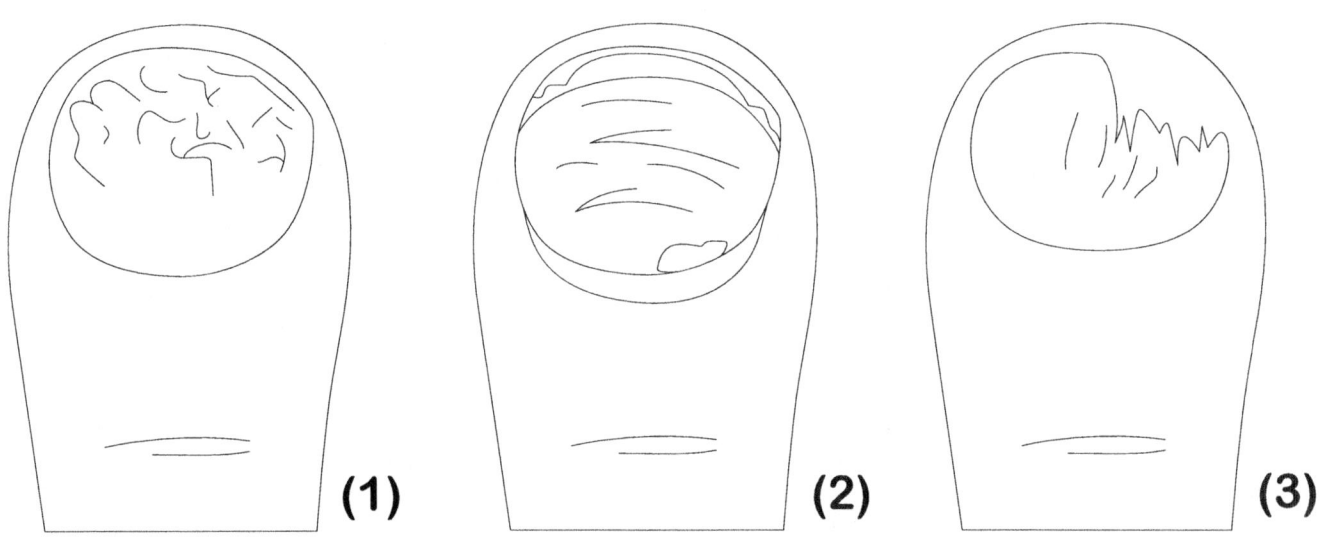

(1) Mold Fungal Infection
(2) Yeast Fungal Infection
(3) Tinea Unguium

Herpes Simplex (Lips/Mouth)

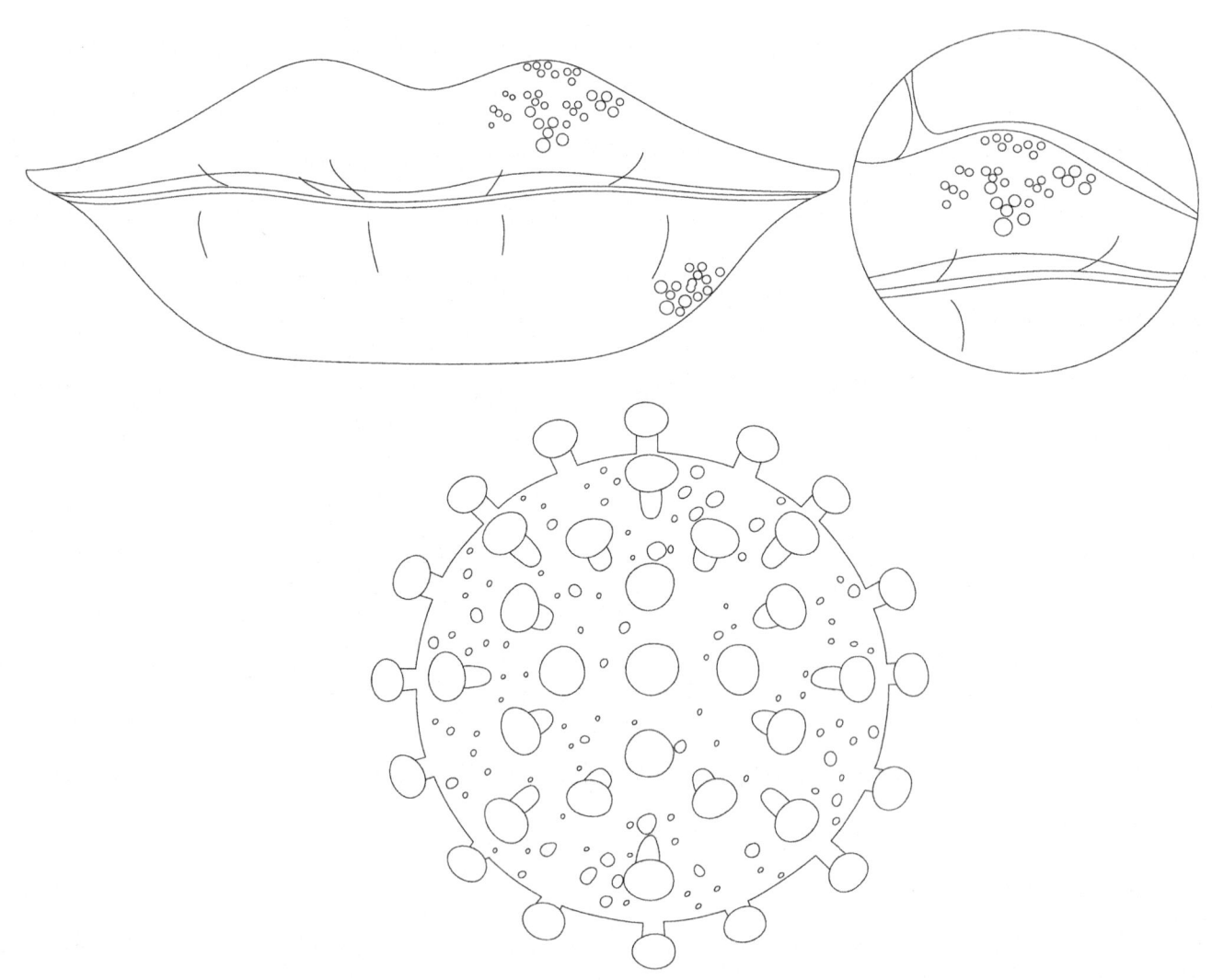

Wart

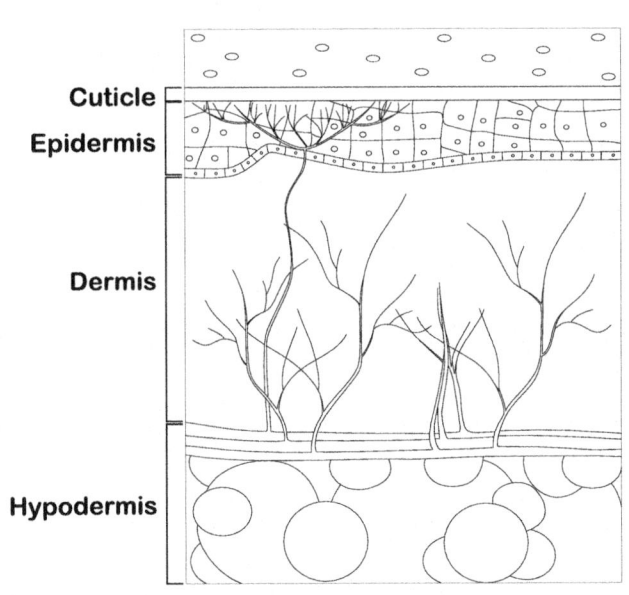
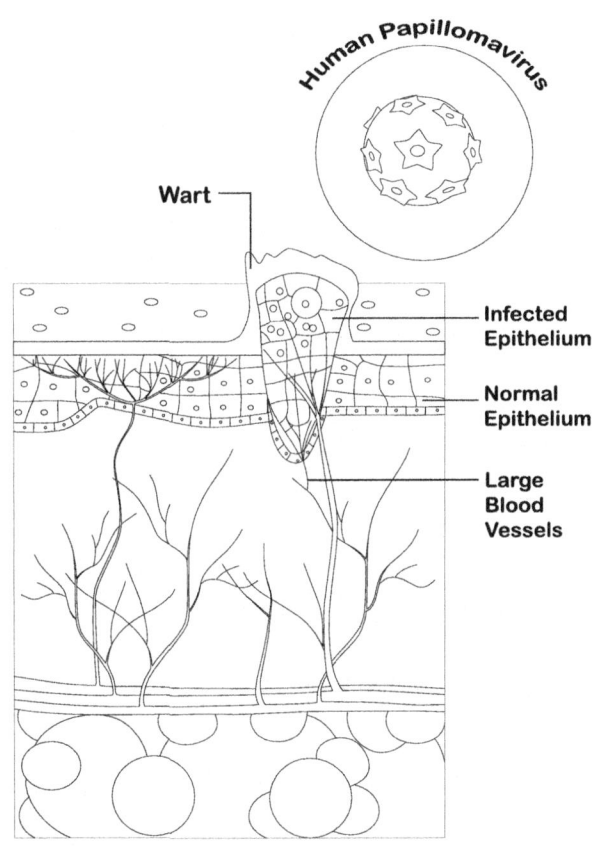

Healthy

Wart

Scabies

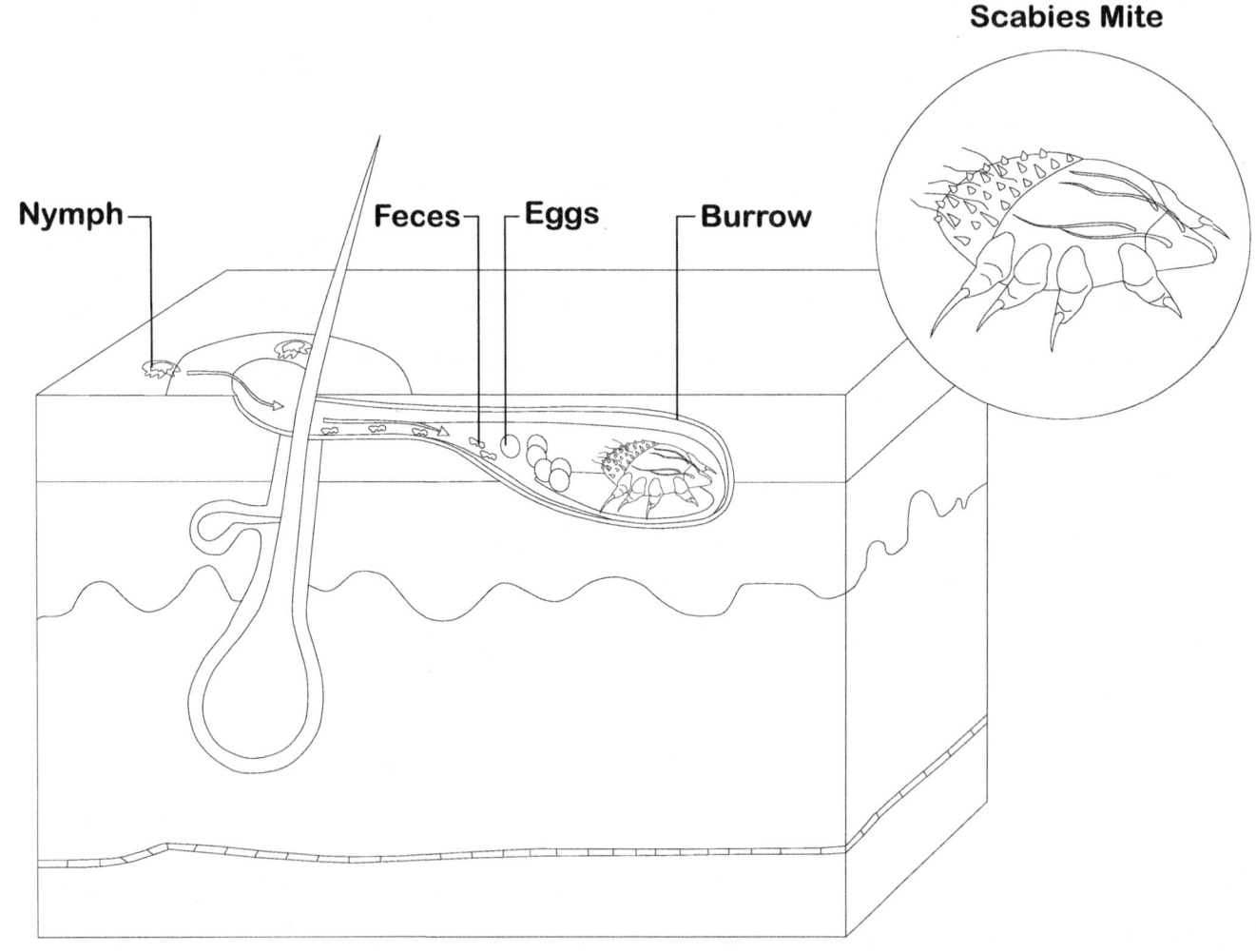

Candidiasis

Oral Candidiasis

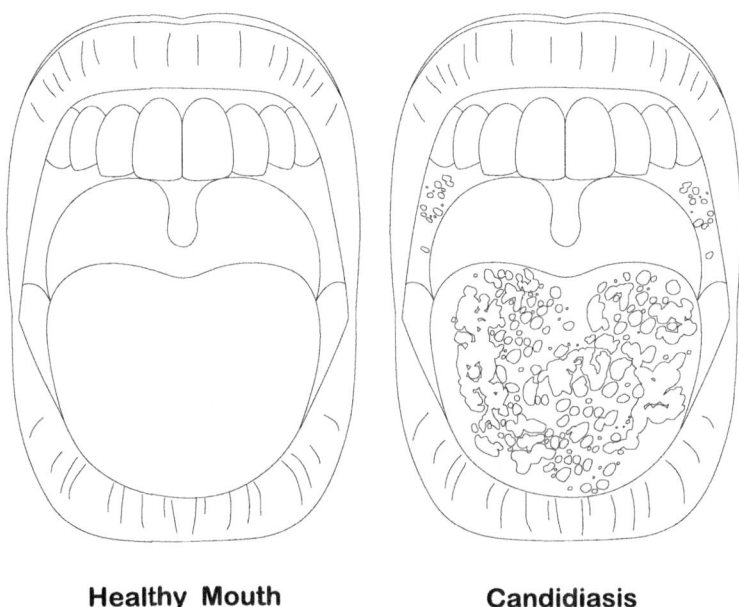

Healthy Mouth   Candidiasis

Vaginal Thrush Candidiasis

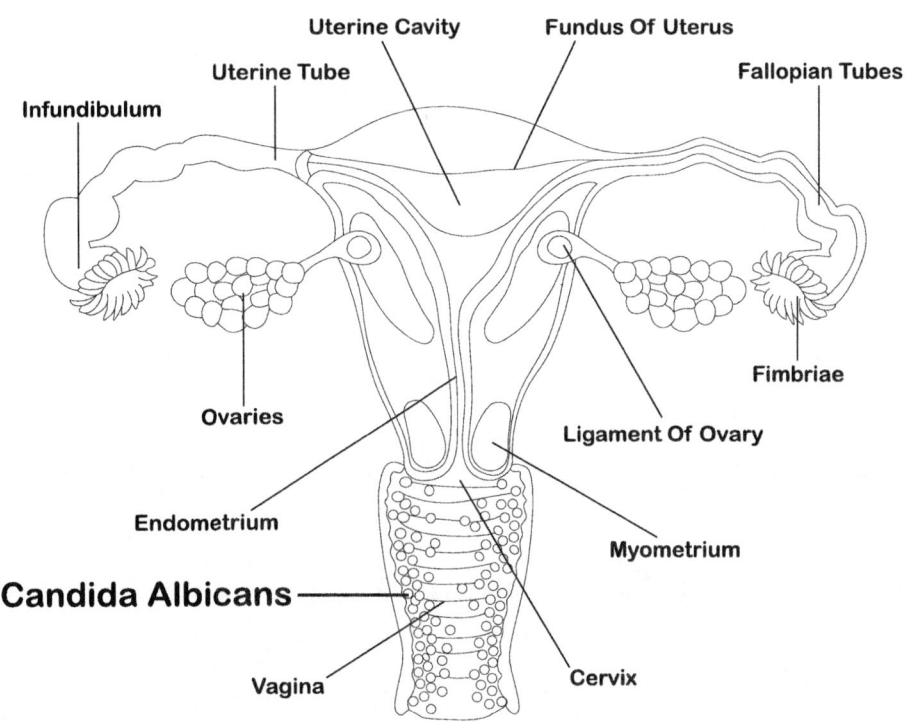

Dental Caries (Tooth Decay)

Stages Of Tooth Decay

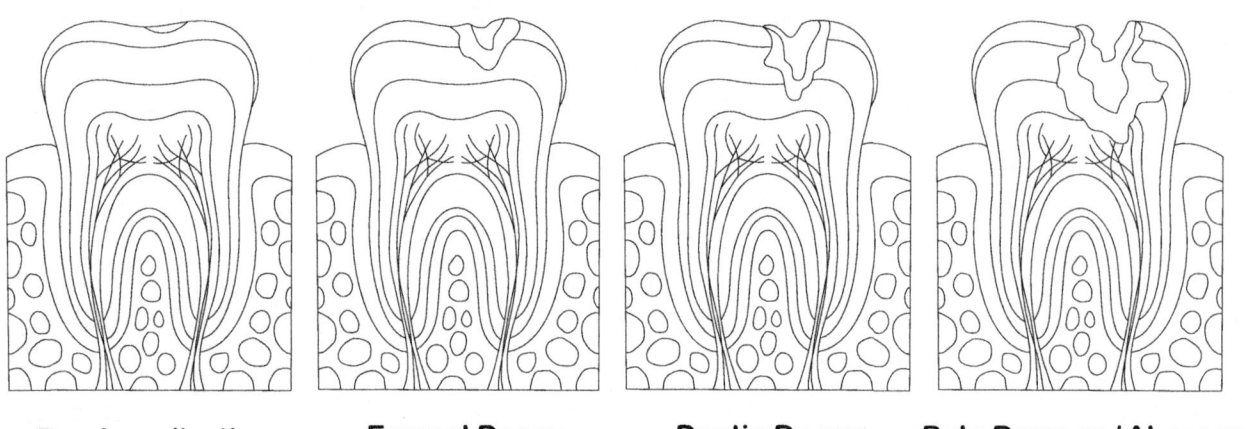

Demineralization | Enamel Decay | Dentin Decay | Pulp Damage / Abscess

Gingivitis

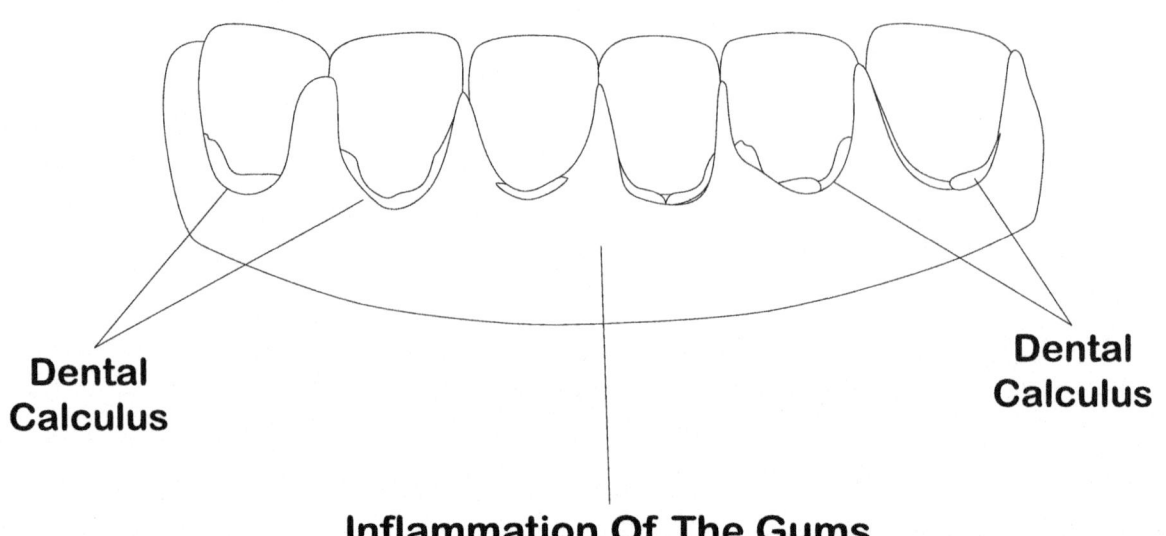

Dental Calculus

Dental Calculus

Inflammation Of The Gums

Periodontitis

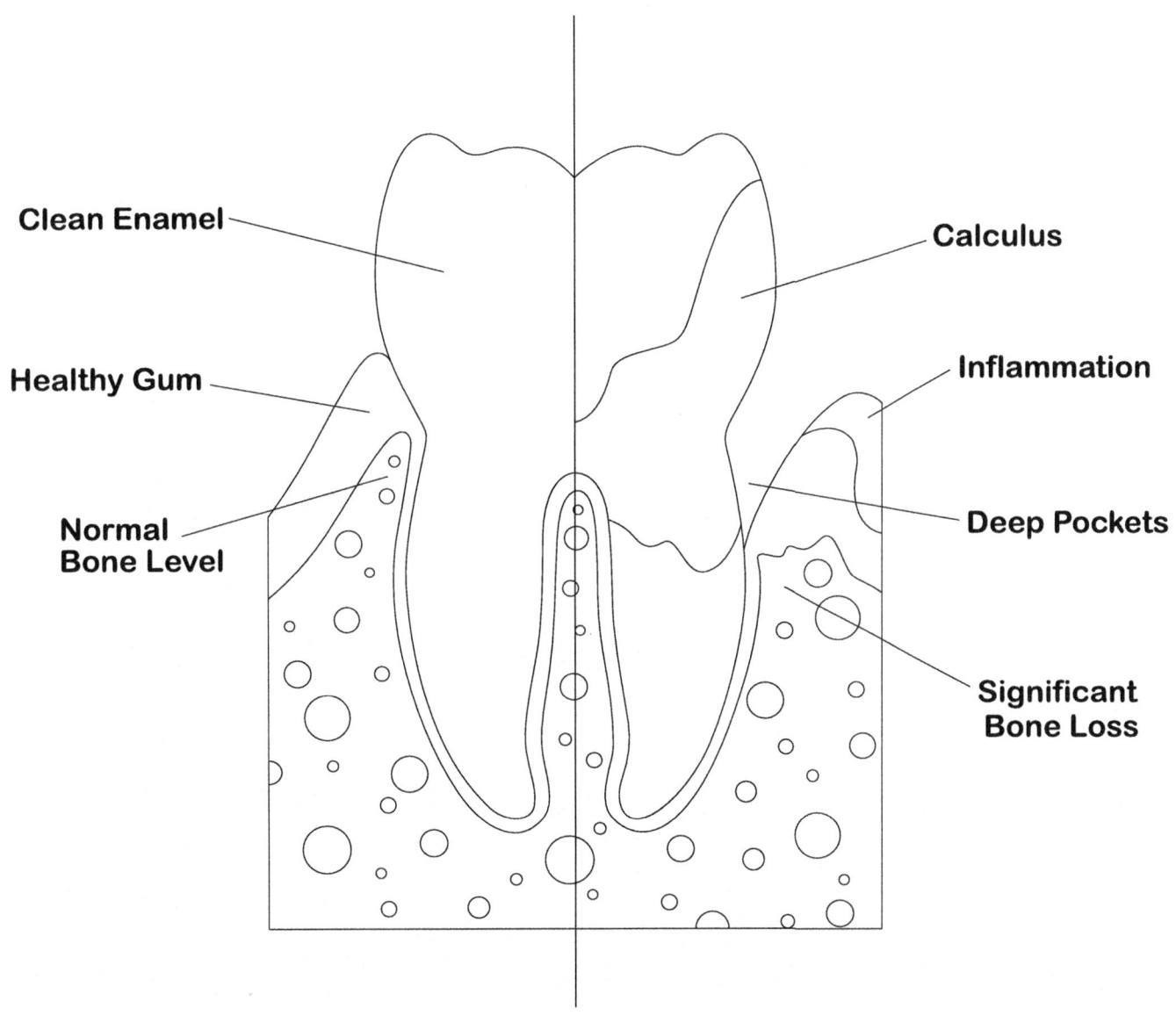

Dental Abscess

Abscess In The Gum

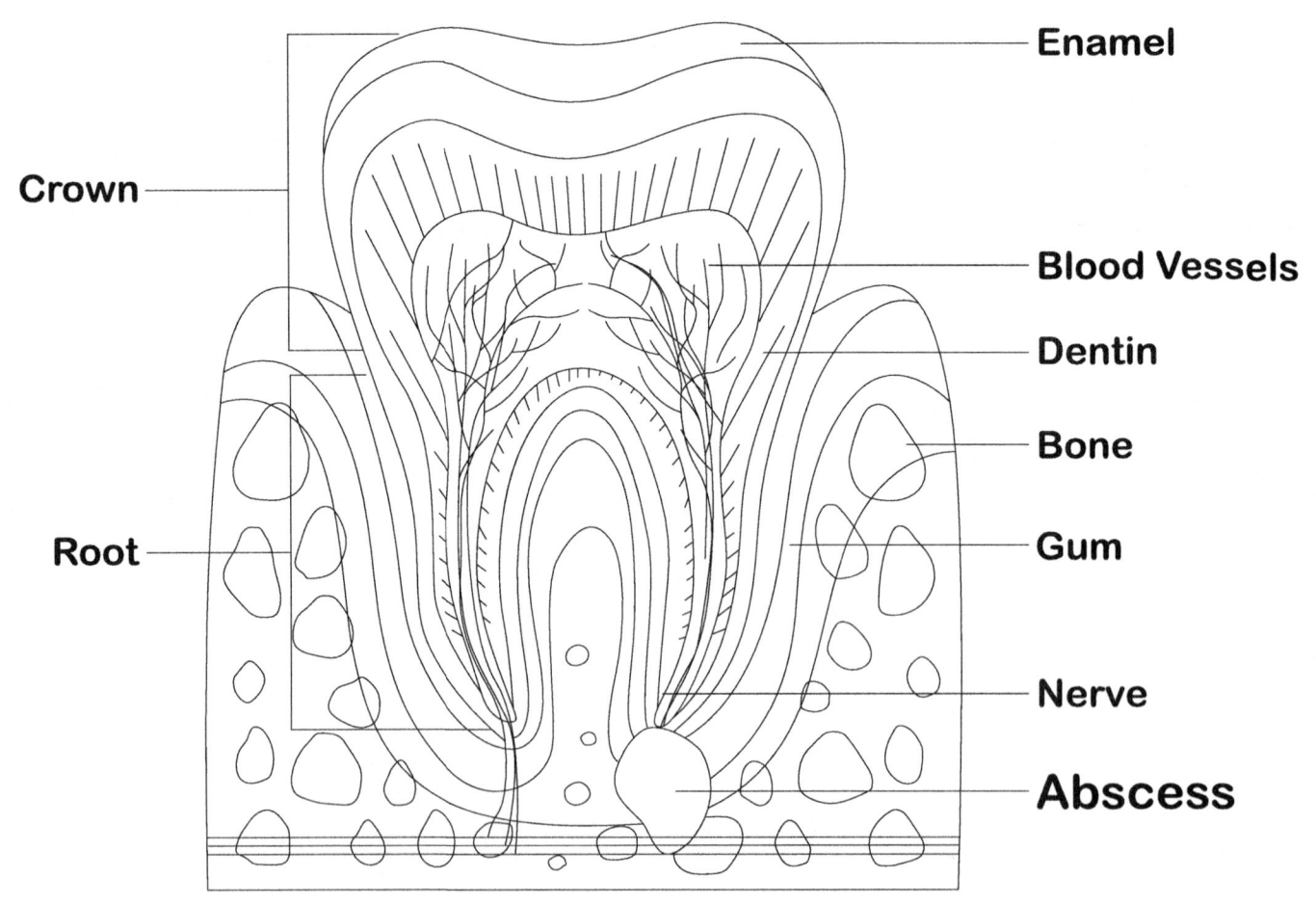

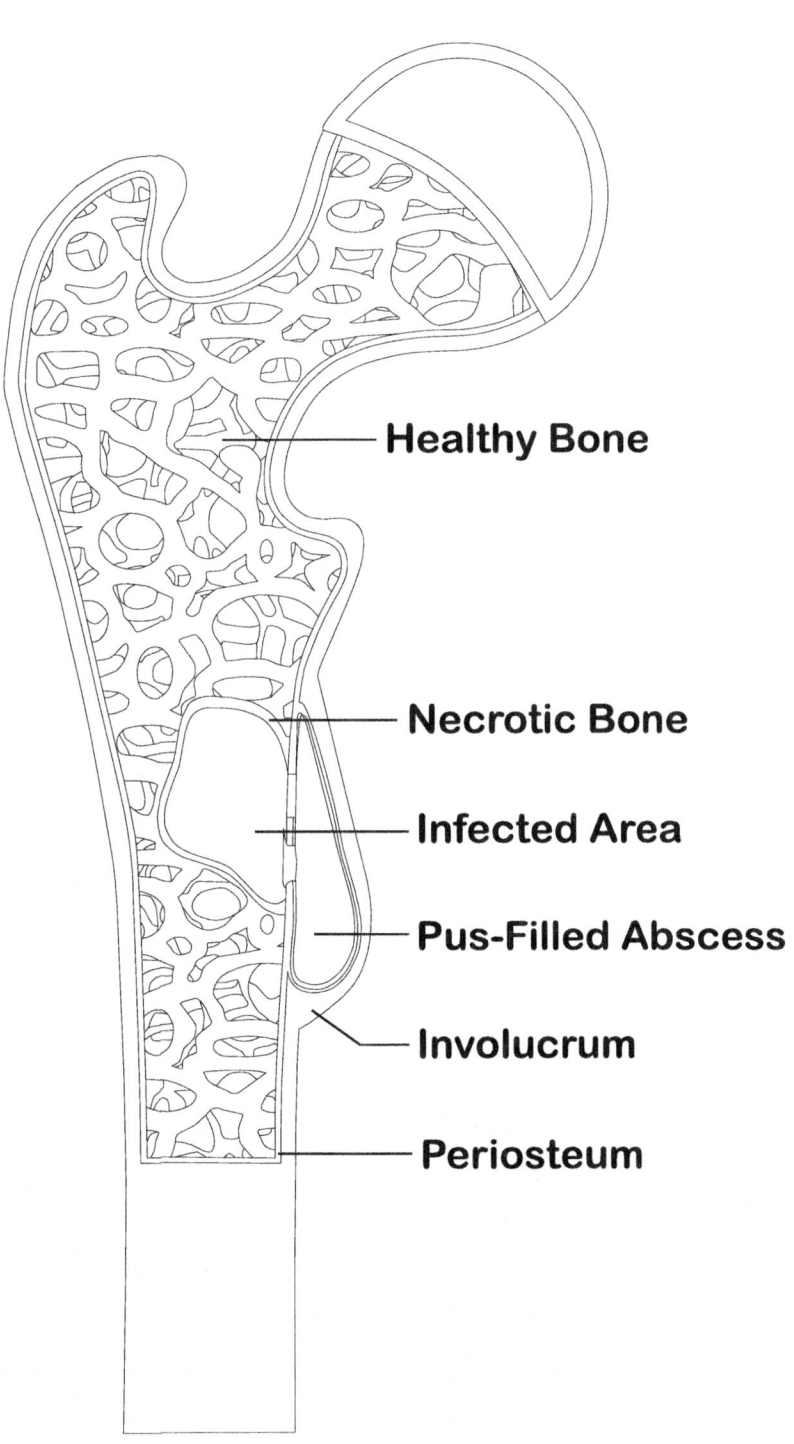

Septic Arthritis

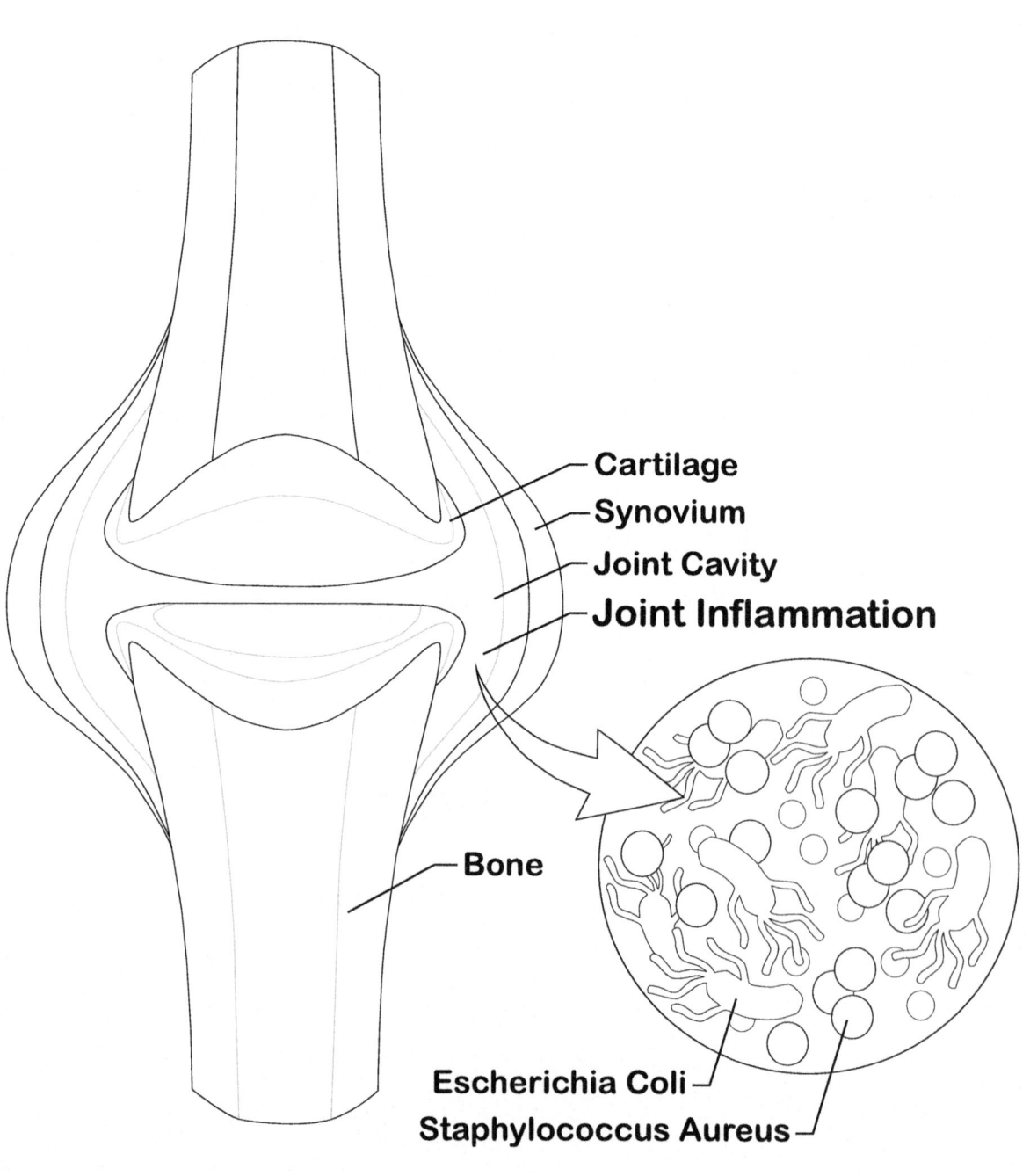

Osteoarthritis

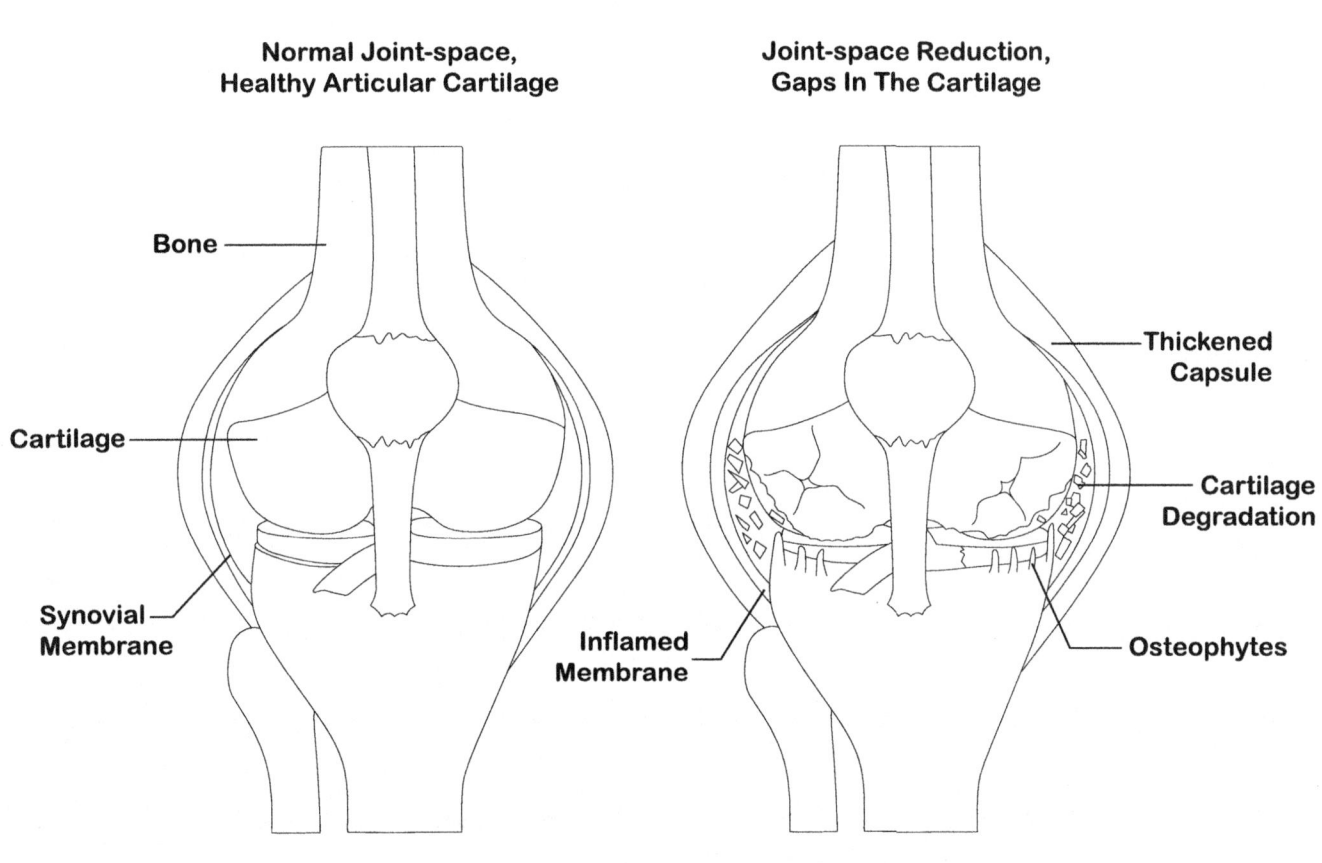

Rheumatoid Arthritis

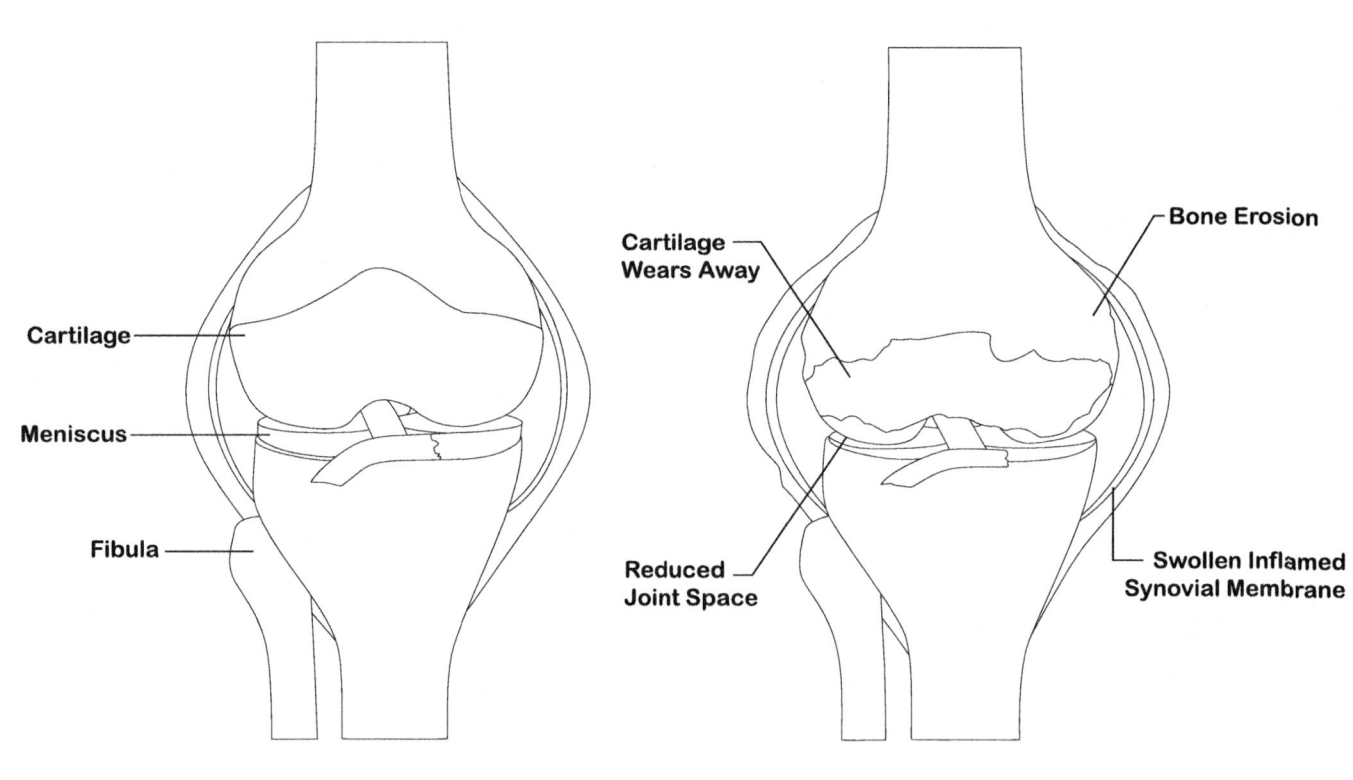

Gout
(Gouty Arthritis)

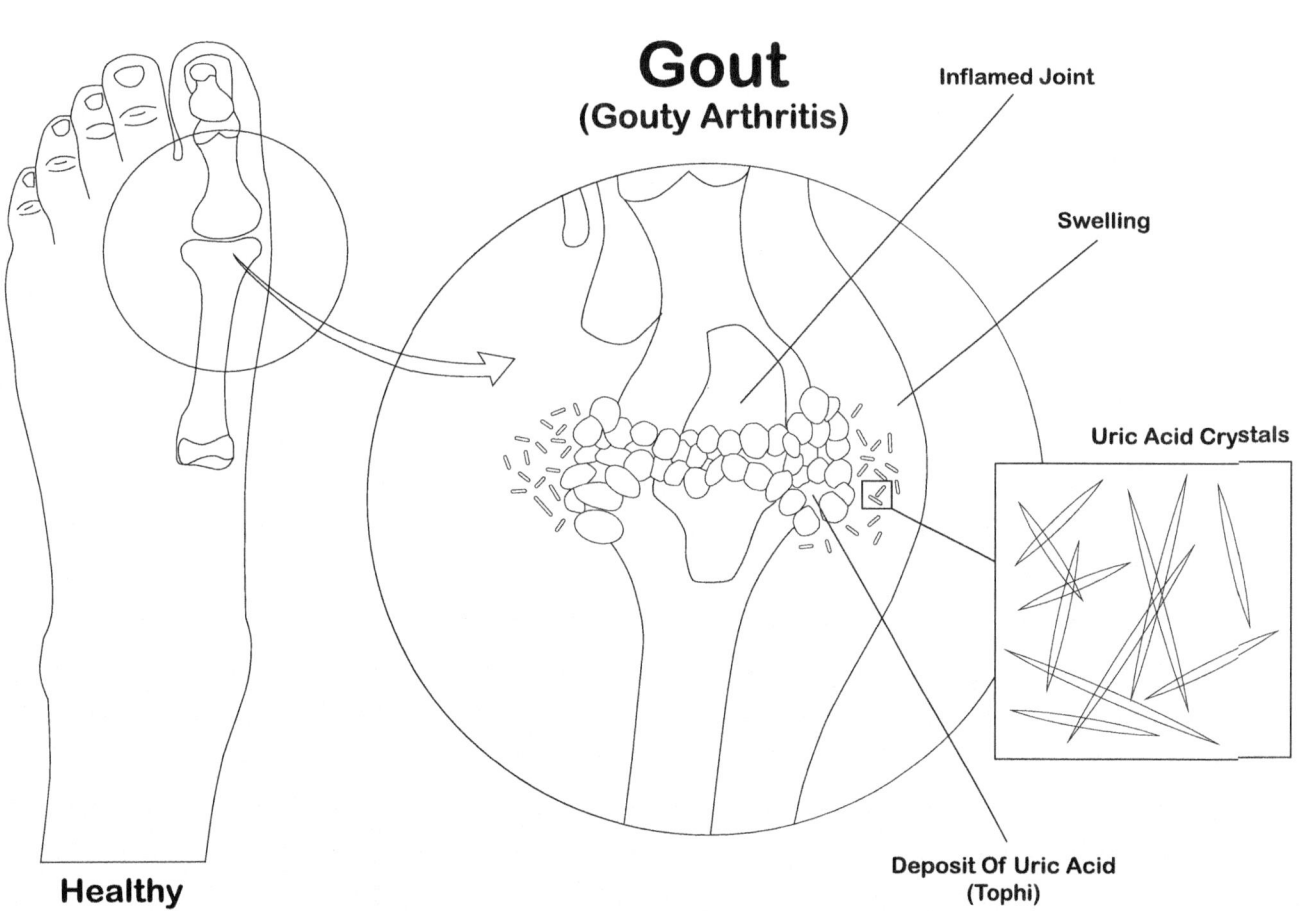

Necrotizing Fasciitis

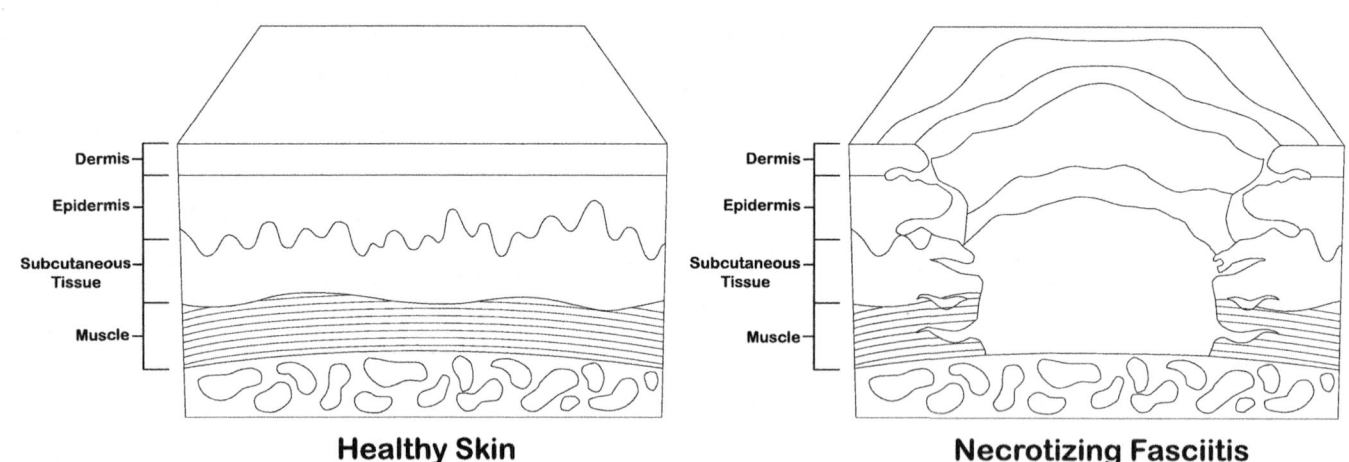

Osteoporosis

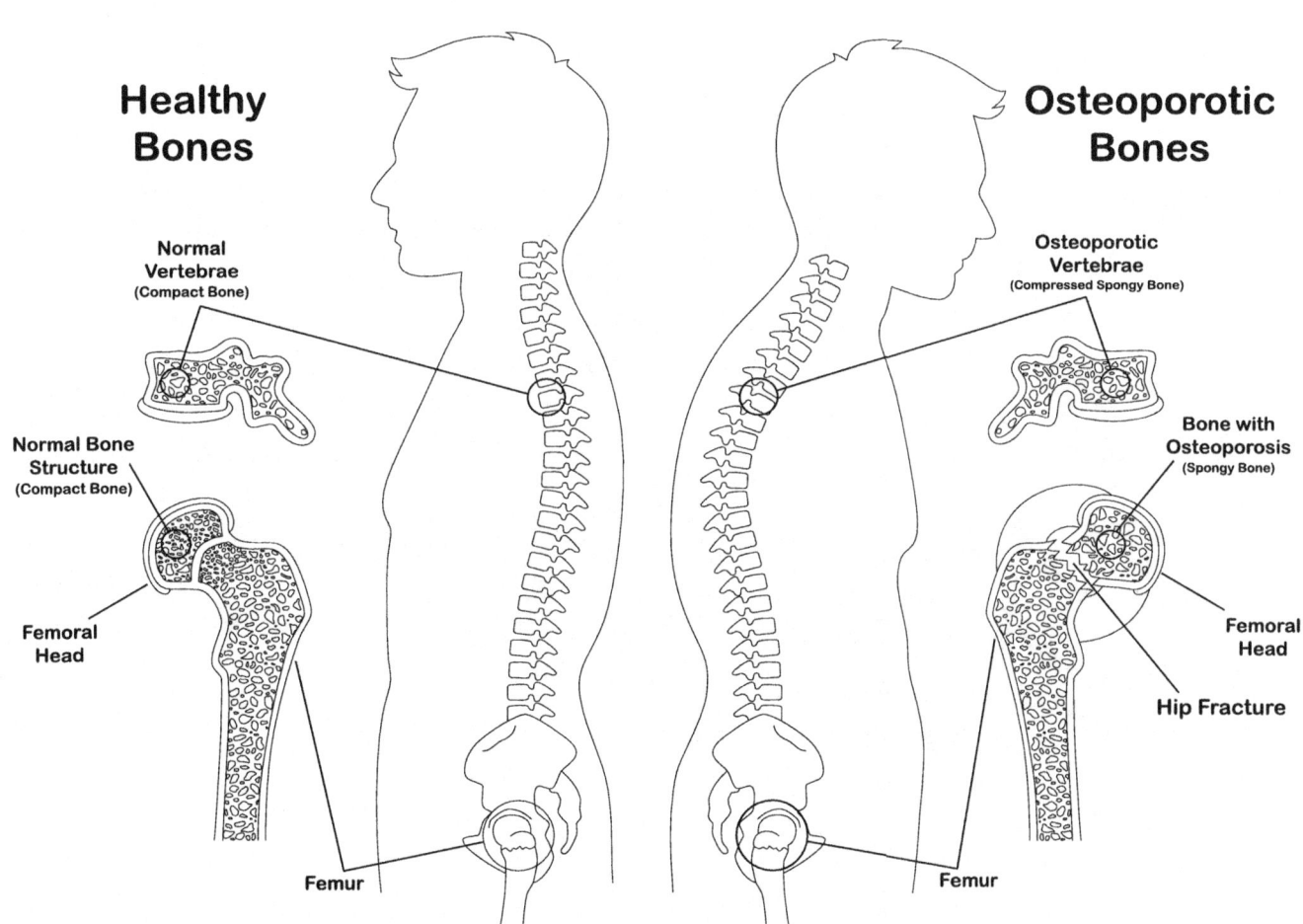

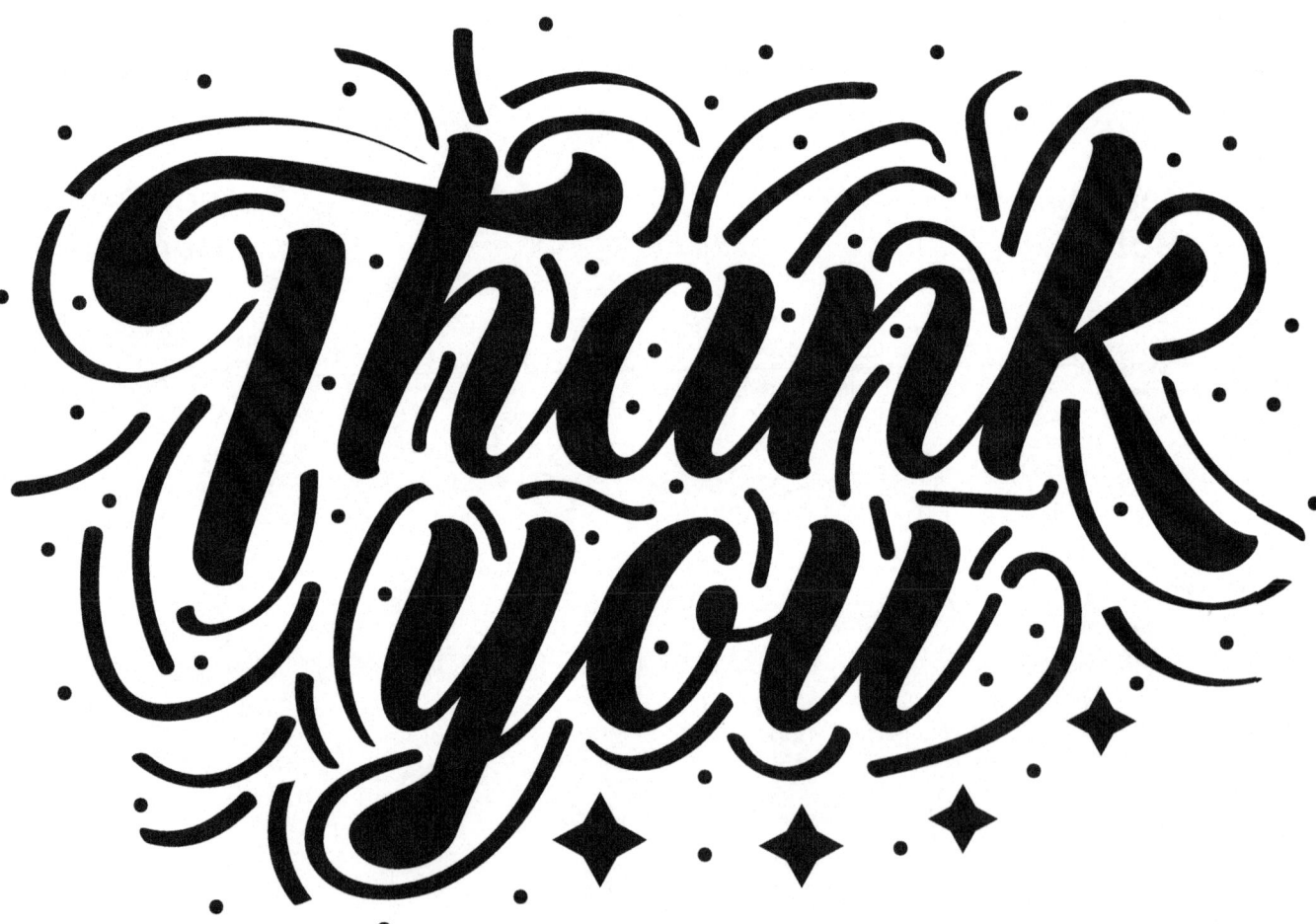

Printed in Great Britain
by Amazon